PATIENT-FOCUSED HYPOTHYROIDISM TREATMENT: A GUIDE FOR PATIENTS AND PRACTITIONERS

TIME-HONORED, CLINICALLY-BASED DOSING FOR AN UNDERACTIVE THYROID

DONNA G. HURLOCK, MD

PHOTO/IMAGE CREDITS
Author Photos: Michael Devaney at Sarasota Photo Studio
Pages 25, 37, 179, 189, 190, 195: Donna G. Hurlock, MD
Page 211: Pixabay
All other photos: Istockphoto

ISBN: 978-1-66787-710-5
Cover design and editing: Mary Shomon
Printed in the USA.
First Edition

Website: https://www.doctorhurlock.com

A CAUTION TO READERS

The publisher and the author are providing this book and its contents in as-is condition and make no representations or warranties of any kind with respect to this book or its contents. The publisher and the author disclaim all such representations and warranties, including but not limited to warranties of healthcare for a particular purpose. In addition, since medical knowledge is constantly changing and expanding, the publisher and the author assume no responsibility for errors, inaccuracies, omissions, or any other inconsistencies herein.

The content of this book is for informational purposes only and is not intended to diagnose, treat, cure, or prevent any condition or disease. You understand that this book is not intended as a substitute for consultation with a licensed practitioner. Please consult with your own physician or healthcare specialist regarding the suggestions and recommendations made in this book. The use of this book implies your acceptance of this disclaimer.

The publisher and the author make no guarantees concerning the safety of application to any individual and the level of success you may experience by following the advice contained in this book, and you accept the fact that results will differ for each individual. The testimonials and examples provided in this book show exceptional results, which may not apply to the average reader, and are not intended to represent or guarantee that you will achieve the same or similar results.

AUTHOR'S NOTE: Throughout the book, where first names are used to identify a patient, these names are pseudonyms to protect patient privacy.

"We look for medicine to be an orderly field of knowledge and procedure. But it is not. It is an imperfect science, an enterprise of constantly changing knowledge, uncertain information, fallible individuals, and at the same time lives on the line. There is science in what we do, yes, but also habit, intuition, and sometimes plain old guessing. The gap between what we know and what we aim for persists. And this gap complicates everything…"

— Atul Gawande, MD,
from "Complications: A Surgeon's Notes on an Imperfect Science"

DEDICATION

This book is dedicated to the thousands of hypothyroid patients who have come from near and far to see me over the past 2+ decades, who have relentlessly searched to find someone who can help them with their many and varied symptoms of hypothyroidism. Their curiosity, patience, and persistence have repeatedly amazed me, despite so many of them previously traveling down so many frustrating paths along the way. I have learned so much from each and every one of my patients and am humbled by the trust they have given me in our mutual pursuit of finding that elusive personal cure. Despite repeated criticism from physicians who seem to worship thyroid stimulating hormone (TSH) like it's a god – while they ignore what their patients are telling them – each success has motivated me to continue to see more patients in hopes of also improving their health and well-being.

And now, during retirement, I hope that this book will help those patients – and patients I have never met – to find the clinical care that they need to be and stay healthy and well. I also hope this book will reach other open-minded physicians, who can incorporate more effective hypothyroidism diagnosis and treatment practices to improve their patients' health and quality of life.

I owe tremendous gratitude to Broda O. Barnes, MD. His writings opened my eyes to a very different way of measuring thyroid function, which was far superior to how I was taught in medical school. His books helped me find a cure for my own hypothyroidism and that of my daughter and allowed me to improve the lives of thousands of patients. And if it weren't for the wise guidance of my medical school classmate, Alan Gaby, MD, twenty-some years ago when I was wearing gloves indoors, constipated, and losing hair like crazy, I would never have learned about Broda Barnes' work.

Finally, I am tremendously grateful to my long-time friend Mary Shomon, a knowledgeable and influential voice in the world of hypothyroidism care, who has taken me under her very experienced wing to edit and produce the final result you are currently reading. Without her help, you would likely not be reading these words at all. Thank you, Mary, for all of your help and encouragement in this book publishing adventure! And thanks also for all you have done for so many years for the hypothyroid community!

CONTENTS

INTRODUCTION

I'm not the first doctor to criticize modern hypothyroidism diagnosis and treatment. In 1976, when I was in medical school, the pioneering Broda Barnes, MD, published his groundbreaking book, *Hypothyroidism, the Unsuspected Illness*. During my medical training, Dr. Barnes' book was never mentioned, but I now consider his work pivotal to understanding the proper way to diagnose and treat hypothyroidism.

I hope this book, inspired by Dr. Barnes' influential work, will add to the vital understanding of hypothyroidism and serve as a useful 'How To" manual for today's practitioners and patients.

Guided by the knowledge I gained from Dr. Barnes – and the experience of working with thousands of women with hypothyroidism – I've learned that no two individuals are hormonally alike. And hypothyroidism manifests itself in many different ways in different people. Consequently, rather than following strict and narrow lab-based guidelines for thyroid replacement, the best results for patients come from individualizing treatment for each patient via careful clinical assessment.

This book offers practical guidance on how to choose a thyroid medication and how much of it to use to replace thyroid hormone in each patient properly. We will also discuss common problems and complicating factors that can occur during this process and how to deal with them – or better yet, how to avoid them.

Again, not every patient fits neatly into a particular diagnostic code box. And no two thyroid patients are the same. Consequently, no "one size fits all" protocol will help all hypothyroid patients get well. Thus, we will continue to need dedicated and caring clinicians willing and able to use their clinical skills to successfully evaluate and manage hypothyroid patients.

Without clinicians who are able to do clinical assessments and see past the misleading laboratory tests, health care for these patients will remain ridiculously complex, expensive, and inefficient. Patients will continue to suffer needlessly, despite taking multiple medications. With more reliance on clinical assessment and much less on laboratory testing, the cost and the quality of care for hypothyroid patients can be dramatically improved. Both have certainly been true in my practice, and I am tremendously thankful for that!

One final note: As a gynecologist, my entire clinical frame of reference has centered on caring for female patients. So please realize that this book describes the management of hypothyroidism in women. That said, having treated hypothyroidism in a few male friends, I have observed that most of their symptoms were the same. Like women with hypothyroidism, the men were often sluggish, struggling with weight gain, and had a depressed mood. There are a few points of departure, however.

For example, the men rarely complained of cold intolerance. And when they had hair loss, they typically accepted it as normal. And the most significant difference was that, as men are often inclined, they rarely went to the doctor to seek help for these symptoms. Instead, they assumed that their symptoms were a normal part of life that they had to accept. So please accept my apologies for my lack of expertise with male patients. That said, it's safe to assume that this book's general approach to diagnosing and managing hypothyroidism will also apply to men.

Patient-Focused Hypothyroidism Treatment

Optimal management of hypothyroidism is an art, and now, in retirement, I feel compelled to pass on the techniques I have learned along the way. I hope my book can help clinicians help their patients and help patients get the best possible care, in the same way that Dr. Barnes' book has helped so many. I hope that at least some physicians will feel validated and continue to practice the true art of medicine, despite the pressures of modern corporate medicine to abandon the art and follow protocols and "best practices" that simply don't serve patients.

I wish you all good health and optimal wellness!

Donna G. Hurlock, MD

PART 1: HYPOTHYROIDISM DIAGNOSIS AND TREATMENT–PAST AND PRESENT

CHAPTER 1: THE HISTORY AND EVOLUTION OF THYROID HORMONE REPLACEMENT

"Beware of false knowledge; it is more dangerous than ignorance."
~ George Bernard Shaw

Fatigue. Depression. Brain fog. Muscle and joint aches. Weight gain. Cold hands and feet. Sleep problems. Low sex drive. Hair loss. Elevated cholesterol. Do any of these symptoms sound familiar? They are actually some of the most common health complaints that plague us today. And billions of dollars – and countless hours – are spent seeking effective treatments and solutions.

The media bombards us with advertisements for products, procedures, plans, nutraceuticals, and pharmaceuticals, all designed to address these issues separately. Pillows, mattresses, sound machines, and more supplements and pills promise to put us to sleep. Energy drinks, triple espressos, and pricey drugs promise to wake us up and keep us awake. "Experts" hawk overpriced miracle supplements, diet programs, and exercise fads to help us lose weight.

And let's not forget the widely-prescribed – and highly profitable – statin drugs to lower cholesterol. (More than a few internists over the years have told me that high cholesterol is so prevalent that "statins should be added to the water supply!")

Wouldn't it be amazing if we could find an easier way to fix these symptoms by identifying the root cause and using that information to create an inexpensive and *effective* solution?

That's why, after decades in medical practice, I am passionate about encouraging practitioners and patients to revisit the metabolic control center of the body – the thyroid gland – to understand why these symptoms are so rampant and learn how to resolve them efficiently!

THE FUNCTION OF THYROID HORMONE

The thyroid gland produces thyroid hormones, whose function is to regulate the metabolic rates of all mammals, including humans. A healthy human or animal thyroid gland produces several hormones, but two are key: thyroxine and triiodothyronine.

The majority of thyroid hormone produced is thyroxine, abbreviated as T4, to indicate that it contains four atoms of iodine. Some consider T4 to be a precursor or storage hormone, and allegedly it has no functional role apart from being converted in the body to T3, which contains only three atoms of iodine. T3 is considered the "active" form of thyroid hormone, and its job is to help activate or drive the various functions within every cell, tissue, gland, and organ system in the body. As noted, most of the T3 in the body is derived from converting T4 into T3, but some T3 is produced and released by a functioning thyroid gland. I'm not entirely convinced that T4 is not an active hormone in the cells, but this is all just theory and is, therefore, not crucial to this discussion.

To help people understand the role of these thyroid hormones, I like to describe them as the "operating system" of the human computer. Your computer needs the "Windows" operating system to run programs like Word or Excel. Similarly, in the body, we require sufficient and functional levels of thyroid hormones as our operating system so that all our individual "programs" – like respiration, digestion, cognition, and such – can run. When we don't have enough thyroid hormone function – a condition known as hypothyroidism – it's like trying to run your computer with a corrupted operating system. Programs get glitchy and don't work well or at all. Instead, your computer body becomes sluggish.

With hypothyroidism, everything slows down, and all our physiologic processes don't work smoothly. The result? Typically, people who are hypothyroid experience fatigue, depression, brain fog, muscle and joint aches, weight gain, cold hands and feet, sleep problems, low sex drive, hair loss, and elevated cholesterol…and many other symptoms. Again…sound familiar?

There *is* an effective way to address these issues. But that knowledge has been relegated to the past for the most part. Why, you ask? Perhaps it's because so many people and corporations (pharmaceutical and non-pharmaceutical) make money selling promises and solutions, and they have a vested interest in keeping it that way. (Ka-ching!)

THE CLASSIC APPROACH TO DIAGNOSING HYPOTHYROIDISM: IDENTIFYING LOW METABOLISM

Going back to the early 20th century, the knowledge of how to diagnose and treat hypothyroidism started with physicians who had a basic knowledge of the natural function of thyroid hormone in the human body. Those were the days when doctors touched patients instead of focusing primarily on their electronic medical records iPads. A physician took a detailed history, asking about symptoms like fatigue, weight gain, cold intolerance, hair loss, depression, and brain fog. A physical examination was also essential. The physician would test reflexes, note a patient's weight and blood pressure, assess the dryness of the skin, evaluate for hair loss, look for puffiness around the eyes and in the hands and feet, and take basal temperatures. After a detailed discussion, careful evaluation of clinical signs, and knowledge of normal human physiology, doctors could make a clinical diagnosis of low metabolism due to thyroid dysfunction and determine that hypothyroidism was the root cause of their patient's symptoms.

This classic approach to diagnosing hypothyroidism served generations of patients and physicians for the first half of the 20th century.

THE CLASSIC APPROACH TO TREATING HYPOTHYROIDISM: CLINICAL WELLNESS AS A GOAL

Since thyroid hormone controls each individual's metabolic rate, it was concluded that thyroid function was inadequate when clinical signs suggested a low metabolic rate. To improve those patients' health, their physicians logically sought to treat them with thyroid hormone replacement, i.e., replacing what was clearly missing based on their physical assessment of their patient. And the goal of treatment was to normalize the metabolism of the individual being treated and relieve all the symptoms of hypothyroidism that were present in each patient.

This was accomplished by starting the patient on a low dose of thyroid hormone replacement. After prescribing a starting dose, the physician carefully adjusted that dose upward – a process called "titration" – until most or all of the patient's symptoms were resolved, without unwanted side effects from overmedication. Back in those days, the dose was usually given three times a day, as many patients found that the efficacy of each dose waned after about 8 to 10 hours.

The dose that relieved the most symptoms and caused no adverse effects was considered the "optimal" dose for each patient. Since the optimal dose of thyroid hormone for each patient varied significantly, a "one size fits all" approach was *not* recommended. Instead, doctors titrated each patient's dose to find the optimal dose.

Later, as blood tests became available around the 1950s, some doctors added a serum cholesterol level as an indirect measure of thyroid function that could help confirm their diagnosis. They knew back then that thyroid function, to a large extent, determined cholesterol levels. When thyroid function was low, cholesterol was usually elevated. And once doctors found the optimal dose of thyroid, they would measure cholesterol again to ensure it had also normalized, which confirmed to them that their dose was indeed adequate.

The bottom line is this: For many decades, physicians – using good old-fashioned logic and reasoning – looked for signs and symptoms of low metabolism and hypothyroidism in order to make a diagnosis. They treated patients with thyroid hormone replacement until hypothyroidism symptoms were safely and satisfactorily resolved and patients felt well! (These patients didn't require a pharmacy full of drugs to treat multiple symptoms. Imagine that!)

THE CLASSIC THYROID HORMONE REPLACEMENT DRUG: ARMOUR THYROID

Thyroid hormone replacement underwent an evolution starting in the late 1800s, when early pioneers like G.R. Murray started administering injections of sheep thyroid extract – which contained natural forms of both T4 and T3 – to their patients.

Doctors soon discovered that oral preparations of animal thyroid extract were also effective, making cumbersome and expensive injections obsolete. The science evolved, and it turned out that porcine (pig) thyroid was even more effective. It was also very inexpensive, as the thyroid glands of pigs were a readily available and otherwise useless by-product of the meat packing industry. The glands were dried (desiccated) into a powder and processed into pills that became a very inexpensive and effective treatment for hypothyroid patients.

Enter Armour and Company, which in 1900 was the largest meat packing company in America. With a near monopoly on porcine thyroid glands, they began manufacturing Armour Thyroid and became the dominant manufacturer of natural desiccated thyroid – also known as NDT – for decades. Over the years, Armour Thyroid went through various owners, but the name stuck. Since the launch of Armour, other brands of NDT – including Westhroid, Nature-Throid, WP Thyroid, and, most recently, NP Thyroid – came onto the market, often costing less than Armour.

Several NDT brands remain on the market today, but to date, none have been formally approved by the FDA. These drugs came onto the market and were being prescribed long before the FDA was even created, so they are considered "grandfathered." They are regulated by the FDA and legal to prescribe. However, they have not gone through the formal FDA approval process because the FDA did not exist when they were first marketed. NDT drugs, therefore, aren't officially "FDA approved." Nonetheless, they are completely legal to prescribe and take for hypothyroidism. (This is not unusual. For reference, many other drugs such as aspirin, acetaminophen, and nitroglycerine existed before the FDA was created and similarly aren't "approved" by the FDA.)

The proportion of T4 to T3 in today's NDT is about 80% T4 and 20% T3. In contrast, the ratio of T4 to T3 in human thyroid hormone is about 94% T4 to 6% T3. Even though NDT has a higher percentage of T3 than human thyroid hormone, NDT remains the closest naturally derived option to replace thyroid hormone in people. However, it is by no means a perfect match for human thyroid since it contains relatively more T3 than most patients usually need.

Generations of hypothyroid patients were successfully treated with Armour and other brands of NDT for many decades.

INTRODUCTION OF "MODERN" MAN-MADE THYROID PRODUCTS AND "MODERN" TREATMENT

A dramatic change in the way hypothyroidism was treated began in the 1960s. I'll add that the change was *not* in a direction that benefits patients. The motivation for this change was, I believe, money. Natural desiccated thyroid is a naturally occurring substance, and thus it can't be patented on its own. Without a patent, the opportunity for a market monopoly and large profit margin was non-existent. At that time, members of the nascent pharmaceutical industry wanted to market a patentable, profitable thyroid product, which excluded NDT. Enter levothyroxine, a synthetic version of the thyroxine (T4) hormone that many people know by its best-known brand name, Synthroid.

Back in 1914, T4 was first successfully isolated from natural desiccated thyroid by Edward Calvin Kendall at the Mayo Clinic in Rochester, NY. Then in 1927, two British chemists, George Barger and Charles Robert Harrington, figured out how to manufacture T4 synthetically without extracting it from NDT. A new drug, levothyroxine, was born.

While the knowledge of how to synthesize levothyroxine has been known since the 1930s, it wasn't until 1949 when Glaxo Laboratories, now known as GlaxoSmithKline, launched the first commercial product of levothyroxine. An effort to popularize levothyroxine for thyroid hormone replacement began at that time when Hart and MacLagan published a review of levothyroxine in the *British Medical Journal* titled "Oral thyroxine in the treatment of myxedema."[1] Since then, levothyroxine has changed hands several times and is currently owned by AbbVie Pharmaceuticals as the branded product Synthroid, which for years had held the lion's share of the levothyroxine market in the US.

Synthroid brand levothyroxine was heavily marketed to patients and physicians as modern and vastly superior to "old-fashioned, out-of-date pig thyroid." Synthroid, after all, was made in a state-of-the-art, clean, high-tech laboratory, while NDT was "a drug made from the insides of an animal that spends all day in the mud."[2]

Along with a push for levothyroxine came a shift to less personalized treatment approaches. Rather than the physician taking a history, doing an exam, and performing a careful evaluation of signs and symptoms, physicians began to rely on laboratory test results. They later outsourced the all-important personal interaction with patients to "physician extenders" like nurses and Physician Assistants. And instead of one-on-one communications with patients, information was increasingly delivered by postcards, mail, third-party phone calls, and, more recently, email and online "portals," leaving patients to figure out and interpret their results and reports on their own. In the past, doctors touched and interacted with patients. Today, they spend time updating electronic medical records on an iPad to make sure their all-important billing codes are justified, ordering lab tests, uploading data to portals, and overseeing their extenders and support staff.

T3 PLUS T4 VERSUS T4 ALONE

Marketing Synthroid to patients and physicians wasn't big pharma's only plan. They also needed to create a reason for doctors to take patients off their NDT and put them on their new, more expensive medication, levothyroxine. Here's where medical education came into the picture. It's well known that pharmaceutical companies can significantly impact what is taught to medical students. And whatever medical students learn often translates into "standard of care" a few years later. Go to any modern-day Continuing Medical Education (CME) meeting and see who the sponsors are. When a drug company makes a large donation to a medical school by endowing a "chair," for example, they influence what is taught and even sometimes get to choose who is doing the teaching. Because the drug industry wanted to shift how doctors treated hypothyroidism, they started to make significant financial contributions to medical schools half a century ago.

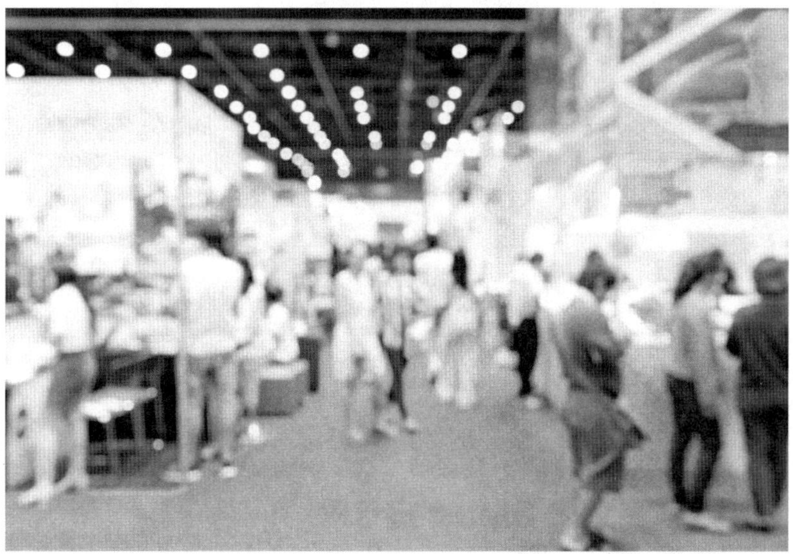

Thanks to pharma's influence on the medical school curricula, the medical establishment quickly declared that hypothyroid patients no longer needed T4 and T3 – namely NDT. A new mantra emerged: *Since the body converts T4 into T3, we only need to replace T4 in hypothyroid patients.* Medical students like myself learned that hypothyroid patients should be prescribed levothyroxine – and only levothyroxine.

No one offered any evidence or even tried to explain how they suddenly knew that every human body *can always* convert T4 to T3 sufficiently and effectively. Or that levothyroxine would work for everyone. But it was repeated over and over, taught in medical schools, and eventually accepted as an established fact.

With a new synthetic T4 to be sold, and a large market of people with hypothyroidism, the behind-the-scenes narrative began to first slander natural desiccated thyroid as old-fashioned, unreliable, and inconsistent, making way for synthetic T4. Then, they sought to replace the old-fashioned and time-consuming method of diagnosing and treating hypothyroidism with clinical findings with a process almost entirely focused on lab tests.

INTRODUCTION OF LABS – THE CORONATION OF THE TSH!

Around this same time, the lab test for thyroid stimulating hormone (TSH), a hormone produced by the pituitary gland, entered the picture. The TSH blood test was introduced to physicians as a new and "more scientific" way to measure thyroid function. The justification was that thyroid levels in the bloodstream are part of a feedback loop, and those thyroid levels in the bloodstream are continually monitored by the hypothalamus and pituitary gland in the brain. When low levels of thyroid hormone are detected, more TSH is released by the pituitary gland.

TSH is a messenger hormone that stimulates the thyroid gland to make more thyroid hormone. The TSH test was based on the idea that when thyroid hormone levels are low, the TSH level goes up to stimulate the gland to produce more hormone. The problem with this approach is that measuring the amount of hormone in the bloodstream does not measure whether or not that hormone is working in the patient's cells.

So, at this point, doctors were being taught – and putting into practice with patients – four unproven theories – all contradicted by scientific facts, as you can see:

THEORY	FACT
Hypothyroid patients only need T4 (the purported precursor/storage hormone) because the body will always effectively convert T4 into T3, the active thyroid hormone.	Healthy thyroid function requires both T4 and T3, and due to variations in absorption rates, enzyme levels, and various other physiologic factors, not everyone can effectively absorb and convert T4 into T3.
The pituitary messenger hormone TSH is a *direct* measurement of thyroid function and metabolic rate.	TSH is a pituitary messenger hormone, *not* a direct measurement of actual circulating thyroid hormones (or whether those hormones are even functional.)
The amount of thyroid hormone in the bloodstream is a *direct* measurement and reflection of thyroid function.	Not all thyroid hormone is available to be used by the cells, and the cells, tissues, and organs of an individual can sometimes be resistant or unable to receive messages from the thyroid hormone in the bloodstream.
The hypothalamic-pituitary-thyroid feedback loop is *always* fully functional.	The hypothalamic-pituitary-thyroid feedback loop can malfunction for many different reasons.

When the hypothalamic-pituitary-thyroid axis is intact, a TSH level is, at best, a surrogate marker for the amount of thyroid hormone in the bloodstream. The TSH level does not, however, directly or even indirectly measure metabolic rate, which is the *function* of thyroid hormone. We still do not have a blood test that directly measures metabolic rate, which would be needed to measure the *function* of thyroid hormone with a blood test.

For most doctors, it was easier to go with the flow of these new ideas from the "experts" at the medical schools and professional societies. As a result, doctors in training and those already in practice quickly fell in line with this dogmatic – and utterly misguided – new paradigm, *apparently without requiring any proof or evidence to support these claims.* They began to revere the TSH test, calling it the "gold standard" test for hypothyroidism. And to this day, they continue to seemingly worship the TSH as the ultimate way to measure thyroid function, even though it doesn't measure metabolism at all.

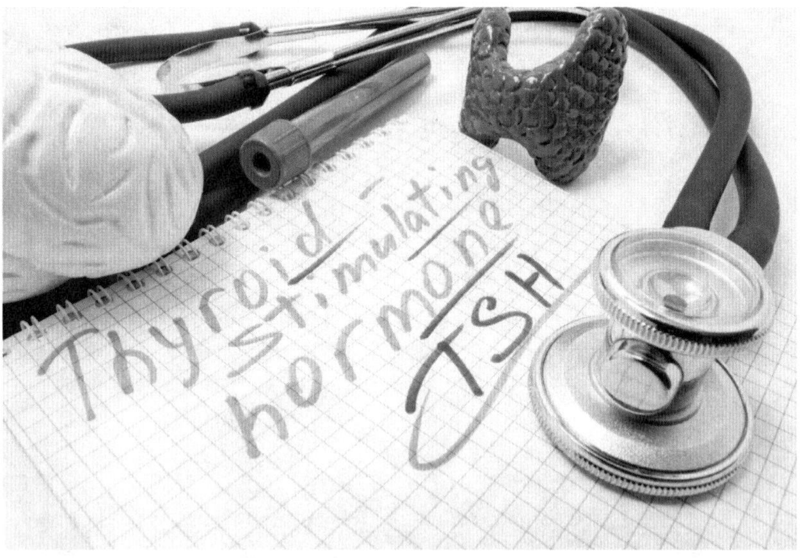

It's no coincidence that the makers of Synthroid, the doctors they enriched, and their friends at the medical schools all supported the idea that the *only* way to diagnose hypothyroidism was to order the almighty TSH test, and the only treatment for hypothyroidism was to "just give T4." Back then, I believed this storyline because I was a young, impressionable medical student, and my exceedingly learned professors and modern textbooks all agreed that this was true. Therefore, it must be the truth, right? (Spoiler: it wasn't!)

THYROID RESISTANCE: LIKE INSULIN RESISTANCE BUT DENIED BY THE EXPERTS

Hormonal physiology is complicated. This is particularly true for large molecules like insulin and thyroid hormone. As discussed earlier, many factors affect both the ability to convert T4 into T3 and absorb thyroid hormone into cells. And, even if the hypothalamic-pituitary-thyroid feedback loop is functioning perfectly – which isn't the case in everyone – the TSH messenger hormone doesn't even reflect the *function* of the thyroid hormone it's indirectly detecting.

All of this rests on a patently false belief: *that the TSH test can measure thyroid function.* This idea is categorically untrue. Measuring thyroid hormone in the bloodstream does *not* reflect whether enough T3, the active thyroid hormone, is actually reaching cells, tissues, glands, and organs to fuel the body's metabolism and function. Yet every textbook published in the past half-century states dogmatically, with no supporting evidence, that TSH measures thyroid function. And how do they know this? "All the experts agree!"

At this point, it's helpful to bring up the example of insulin. Suppose a physician actually measures the amount of insulin in the blood of Type 2 diabetics. In that case, they will find that there is usually enough – or even too much – insulin in the bloodstream. However, that insulin isn't doing its job to move sugar out of the bloodstream. As a result, blood sugar levels become abnormally elevated. High blood sugar in the presence of sufficient insulin is commonly referred to as insulin resistance, which means that the tissue appears resistant to the effects of the available insulin. We understand this concept because we can measure the amount of insulin in the bloodstream *and* blood sugar, allowing us to evaluate the *effectiveness* of insulin. Blood sugar testing tells us whether the insulin is *functional.* As a result, endocrinologists rely on blood sugar levels to guide treatment instead of measuring the amount of the hormone insulin. Smart move on their part, and lucky for their patients.

If they instead used insulin levels to determine their treatment, most of their diabetic patients would go untreated or undertreated and would develop dangerously high blood sugar levels. A patient could be in a diabetic coma and still have plentiful insulin, so the diagnosis would be missed if it weren't for the fact that endocrinologists have universally accepted the concept of insulin resistance. Thankfully, the endocrinologists have figured that out!

Inexplicably, they haven't applied the same understanding to hypothyroidism. They continue to rely on the TSH test to measure thyroid function, ignoring the fact that TSH only indirectly measures the amount of thyroid hormone as seen by the pituitary gland. Still, it doesn't measure the *function* of thyroid at all. In contrast, assays of blood sugar *do measure the function* of insulin. Borrowing from the language of diabetes, these patients have "thyroid resistance." Like a person with diabetes who has *enough* insulin – but has sky-high blood sugar – these hypothyroid patients with a normal TSH level have *enough* thyroid hormone. Their hormone is not effective, however, so the metabolism remains sluggish.

After decades of medical practice treating thousands of hypothyroid patients, I found that most hypothyroid patients have some degree of thyroid resistance. Their "normal" TSH masks the diagnosis. Unfortunately, there's no way that the TSH test can identify thyroid resistance. The hypothalamus and pituitary gland cannot measure our overall metabolic rate to decide how much TSH to make. Do the hypothalamus and pituitary gland know if hands are cold, hair is falling out, skin is dry, or a person is constipated? Can they tell if we are depressed, achy, or if our brain function seems missing in action? And after thyroid treatment starts, can the hypothalamus and pituitary gland tell if hands or feet have warmed up, hair has stopped falling out, bowel movements have become regular, or we are focused, feeling good and happy? *Of course not!*

The TSH test simply can't tell if thyroid treatment relieves the symptoms that brought a patient to the doctor in the first place because it doesn't measure metabolic rate, and it doesn't measure whether symptoms are present or not. It never has, and it never will.

Sadly, for half a century, we've been erroneously taught by myopic experts in endocrinology that as long as their "gold standard" TSH test level is normal, the patient is well. These same endocrinologists acknowledge insulin resistance and would never base their decisions for their diabetic patients on insulin levels. Yet, they rarely, if ever, acknowledge thyroid resistance. They even refer to TSH, T3, and T4 tests as "thyroid function tests," when those tests no more measure thyroid function than an insulin level measures a diabetic's clinical status.

This is a massive problem because almost all doctors today use the TSH level to diagnose hypothyroidism and measure the so-called success of hypothyroidism treatment. Over the last 50 years, this is what experts have been saying and teaching in medical school. Whatever dose of thyroid medication yields a TSH level that falls into the "normal" reference range is considered the optimal dose. And the biggest failure of all? When today's endocrinologists see their hypothyroid patients for follow-up, and the TSH is now in the normal range, the patient is declared to be "cured," even if all the patient's symptoms are still present!!! No wonder many of their patients are so frustrated and eventually seek doctors like me for a different approach!

These doctors stubbornly refuse to open their eyes and ears to see that many patients have symptoms that persist – even when the TSH is normal. As a result, the TSH test result now determines the doses given to the patient. Clinical wellness is often not a factor, and many patients remain undiagnosed. In many cases, those who are treated remain underdosed because the doses prescribed to normalize the TSH level are almost always inadequate to achieve real clinical wellness.

A patient may be exhausted, depressed, cold, constipated, having sleep problems, and gaining weight despite regular exercise and a strict low-calorie diet. But when the TSH is normal, most modern doctors cannot put all these clues together to diagnose hypothyroidism because "the thyroid function tests are normal!" So, doctors tend to blame their patients' symptoms on other conditions. "You're tired because you have kids, and you work." "You're gaining weight because you overeat and need to exercise more." "You're losing hair because you're stressed."

Hypothyroid patients end up with referrals for sleep studies for fatigue, gastric bypass for obesity, and prescriptions to treat everything from high cholesterol to depression. Other patients are shipped off to specialists to be diagnosed with conditions such as chronic fatigue syndrome, fibromyalgia, ADHD, and narcolepsy. More drugs are prescribed – an SSRI for their depression, a sleeping pill for disrupted sleep, a statin for their high cholesterol, and perhaps a little Adderall for their inability to focus. As you can imagine, this approach quickly becomes quite complex and costly and usually yields limited benefits.

However, this convoluted process is *excellent* for business if you're a pharmaceutical company, own a sleep center, hold a patent for a CPAP machine, or are a bariatric surgeon doing gastric bypass surgeries for cash. I suspect profit is the primary reason there is so much pressure from the medical/pharmaceutical industry to maintain the fiction that thyroid blood tests somehow measure thyroid function. In my opinion, the idea that TSH measures thyroid function turns out to be a very profitable hoax and one that is grossly unfair to hypothyroid patients.

HOW STUDIES ARE MANIPULATED

When patients do their own research and ask their physicians for a trial of NDT, the doctor usually responds: "Why would you want to take that old-fashioned, out-of-date stuff?" Or patients are told that "NDT is inconsistent and unreliable; each batch is different." (This false argument is particularly amusing since the FDA has recalled Synthroid for poor quality and potency problems far more frequently than NDT.) The misinformation about NDT is widespread. Some doctors even believe that NDT isn't a prescription drug or is off the market entirely. Public Citizen's *Worst Pills* report even erroneously disseminated the information that NDT was an "over-the-counter supplement." (Hint: It's not. NDT has *always* required a doctor's prescription!)

As mentioned earlier, after levothyroxine products began to be aggressively marketed as an alternative to NDT in the mid-1900s, a growing bias against the need for and use of T3 started to appear in the literature. Again, if they could convince physicians that patients only needed T4 replaced, that cleared the path for levothyroxine to steal market share from Armour Thyroid.

A perfect example of this anti-Armour thyroid, anti-T3 bias is seen in a paper published in January 2018 in the *International Journal of Clinical Practice* by Drs. Hennessey and Espaillat.[3] They claimed that their goal was to review the literature to once and for all determine whether T3 should be added to T4 when treating hypothyroidism. Displaying their inherent bias, they lamented that "there remains a persistent concept that addition of T3 has a role in the treatment of hypothyroidism, that is, to improve persistent symptoms." Their goal was clearly to show that T3 was not useful in treating hypothyroid patients.

They cherry-picked studies to prove their point, leaving out those over 10 years old and those showing the benefits of adding T3 to T4. Their bizarre justification for this exclusion of data was the following: "Because older research has been well summarized," all the older studies, including all the original data comparing Armour and Synthroid, were excluded from their search. In addition, articles showing the benefit of adding T3 to T4 published around 2000 to 2005 were conveniently excluded by their arbitrary 10-year cut-off. Then they excluded any review articles, apparently to ensure that they would not have to include any findings of the older literature that might be included in those review articles.

Despite their meticulous exclusion of studies that would have disproven their desired outcome, they *still* found the benefit of adding T3 in about a quarter of the studies that they did review. No studies showed harm from adding T3. Nevertheless, the researchers dishonestly concluded that "there is no reproducible clinical evidence to support the efficacy of LT4/LT3 over LT4 alone." They went on to recommend "T4 monotherapy as the treatment of choice" and recommended against the routine addition of T3 to levothyroxine or use of natural desiccated thyroid." (How they made that last conclusion is anyone's guess since *none* of the studies they included in their review even used NDT!)

The illogical nature of their conclusions was perplexing until I read the disclosure information. Both authors were on the payroll of AbbVie Pharmaceuticals, the current owner of Synthroid brand levothyroxine. In fact, AbbVie *funded* the study. So, this scientific study was, in my opinion, a marketing piece produced by the makers of Synthroid.

Even more fascinating is that in recent years, the FDA appears to be unfairly targeting many of the smaller manufacturers of NDT drugs for unusually intensive monitoring and enforcement and has already forced several brands off the market, potentially for good. At the same time, the FDA is seemingly leaving Armour Thyroid alone. Suspicious? I suspect it's because a few years ago, Armour Thyroid was acquired by global pharmaceutical giant AbbVie, the same company that makes Synthroid.

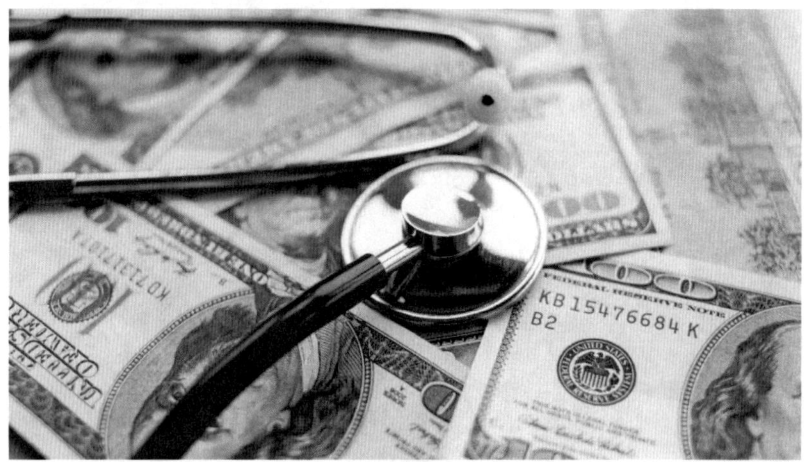

Since that acquisition, it appears to me that AbbVie has taken advantage of Armour's name recognition and dominant market position. At the same time, AbbVie mounted a successful campaign to get the FDA to designate NDT as a "biologic" drug, which occurred in September of 2022. It's likely that the FDA's next step will be to require that NDT go through the formal approvals process reserved for biologic drugs. This process is also so daunting and cost-prohibitive that it could potentially force the few remaining competitive NDT products – all made by smaller manufacturers – out of the market entirely. (Of course, AbbVie already manufactures several of the most expensive biologics on the market, like Humira, Rinvoq, and Skyrizi, and has teams of experienced scientists and overpaid lobbyists who could ensure that Armour sails through the FDA's usually rigorous and expensive approvals process.)

It's all a win-win for AbbVie because the FDA's approval of Armour as a biologic drug could leave the company with a near monopoly on NDT drugs – complementing their dominance in the levothyroxine market. They would also be in a position to significantly raise the price of Armour! It's always about the money!

DOSES NEEDED TO CURE VERSUS DOSES NEEDED TO NORMALIZE THE TSH

Useful Drugs[4] was a guide published a century ago by the American Medical Association that described most or all of the drugs available at that time, including standard dosing practices. (*Useful Drugs* was later replaced by the modern *Physician's Desk Reference* or PDR.) In the 1923 edition of *Useful Drugs*, the usual starting dose of Armour Thyroid was listed as 1 grain (60 mg) taken three times a day (a total of 3 grains). That would be about equal to a total of 300 mcg of levothyroxine. It then stated that patients rarely needed to exceed more than 10 grains (600 mg of Armour) per day to achieve clinical wellness. (For reference, 1 grain of NDT is 60 mg, and 1 grain of levothyroxine is 100 mcg.)

In contrast, the standard dose of levothyroxine currently prescribed by today's endocrinologists ranges from about 50 mcg to 150 mcg, taken once daily. In grains, that would equal ½ to 1½ grains daily. So, the starting dose of 3 grains of thyroid in 1923 was twice as much as the usual highest dose of levothyroxine prescribed by today's endocrinologists. And the highest dose commonly used in 1923 – 10 grains – is about seven times the largest dose commonly used today!

Why is there such a vast difference? It's because the goal of treatment changed back in the 1960s. Before that time, the goal of treatment was clinical wellness: safely relieving the patient's hypothyroidism symptoms. The patient was given whatever dose was required to resolve their symptoms without causing overdose symptoms.

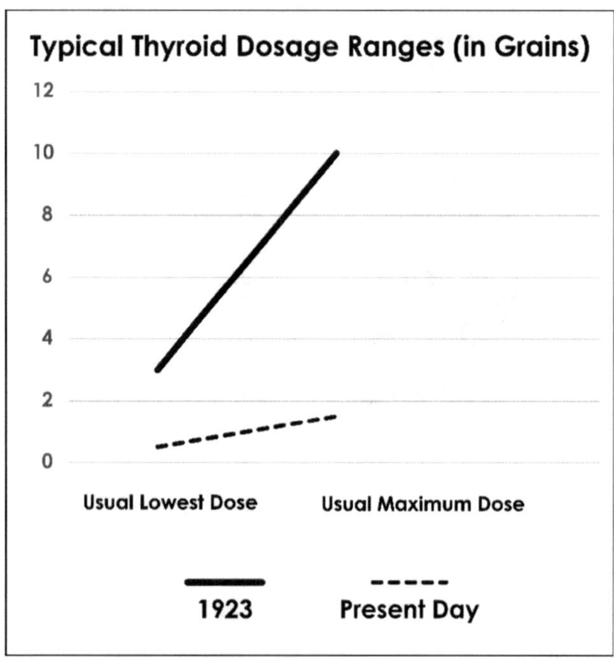

After the introduction of the TSH test in the 1960s, this practice gave way to the new goal: a TSH level in the normal range. However, the dose required to normalize the TSH level in most people is quite small. Moving away from clinical wellness and towards TSH normalization in the 1960s resulted in a massive reduction in the commonly used doses of thyroid. Is it any wonder that modern hypothyroidism treatment doesn't work well in relieving patients' symptoms?

Worse yet, patients with many hypothyroid symptoms –whose TSH is still normal – will frequently remain undiagnosed and untreated! I've often said that a patient could present to the emergency room on a stretcher, entirely bald, 400 pounds, suicidally depressed, wrapped in layers of blankets on a hot day, in a myxedema coma with a pulse of 50, and if the TSH comes back as "normal," a diagnosis of hypothyroidism won't even be considered! Sadly, I've seen patients in my office who have been almost that sick and previously seen multiple other specialists who had been treated exactly that way.

MEASURE THE *FUNCTION* OF THYROID, NOT THE *AMOUNT* OF THYROID!!!

I have found that the best way to diagnose and treat a hormone disorder is the old-fashioned way: *measure the thyroid hormone's function and effectiveness, not the amount of thyroid hormone!* Since we don't have a blood test that measures the patient's metabolic rate, we need to carefully assess the individual patient's clinical signs and symptoms and how those symptoms change with dose changes, always observing for any signs of overdose. The current lab-based system is yielding widespread misdiagnosis and mismanagement of hypothyroidism. And millions of undiagnosed or inadequately treated patients are forced to live with a lifetime of poor health. But hey, they have "normal" TSH levels, so it's all good, right? Wrong!

Let me say it again, plainly and clearly. When diagnosing and treating hypothyroidism, the classic, time-tested way is *better.*

Instead of relying on TSH, a test with almost no direct relationship to hypothyroidism *symptoms*, we need to use careful clinical assessment to diagnose and manage hypothyroidism.

Further, instead of treating all patients with only T4 and defining success only by the TSH level, we should feel free to use *all* the thyroid tools available to us, synthetic T3, T4, and NDT, and safely give enough medication to resolve the symptoms that each individual patient is experiencing. And we should accept the fact that the needs of individuals are very variable, and different patients will respond differently to each product. No one product is "best" for all patients.

Patients don't go to the doctor with the goal of "normal" TSH levels. They go with the goal of getting rid of symptoms and feeling better. If you're a patient who shares that goal, here's my advice: Be persistent! Don't give up on finding a physician to help you feel better. Hopefully, you'll find someone who focuses on clinical outcomes rather than just on lab tests, someone who will finally hear you…and help you. And if you have an open-minded physician who is willing to try but not sure how to do it, you might want to recommend that they read this book.

I also have a message to fellow practitioners: consider adopting this approach, which I explain more fully in this book. Be brave enough to break free from the old TSH dogma and adopt a new approach: Treatment of hypothyroidism should focus on normalizing your patient's metabolic rate and safe relief of their symptoms, *not* on normalizing TSH values!

WHY IS THERE LITTLE INTEREST IN THE PREVENTIVE BENEFITS OF THYROID HORMONE?

In addition to resolving existing clinical signs and symptoms, optimal thyroid hormone treatment has many preventive health benefits. Part 2 of this book outlines the many physiologic systems that are profoundly affected by a lack of thyroid hormone and the many serious, debilitating, and even life-threatening conditions that can be prevented with optimal thyroid treatment. Why is there so little interest among physicians and researchers in these benefits?

Again, what used to be known and understood is no longer known. This is very similar to our understanding of estrogen replacement over the past two decades. All of the literature from the 1970s through the 1990s demonstrated that, when correctly done, hormone replacement therapy (HRT) lowered cholesterol and prevented heart disease. Before the 2002 publication of the Women's Health Initiative (WHI) findings, most clinicians accepted the conclusions of the multiple studies that demonstrated the many benefits of HRT.

But that knowledge went missing. Today, the commonly held and incorrect belief is that hormone replacement is categorically dangerous and has no benefits beyond temporary symptom relief. What used to be the truth is no longer the truth. Do you think the mysterious disappearance of information showing cardiovascular benefits achieved from replacing inexpensive estrogen has anything to do with the appearance of statin drugs on the market in the late 1980s? If you can normalize cholesterol and reduce heart disease with relatively inexpensive HRT – or thyroid hormone for that matter – no one would ever need to buy a statin drug. If most menopausal women were on HRT and adequate thyroid (when required), they would have little need for profitable statins.

In this day and age, cardiovascular disease is the most common cause of mortality in the US. Comprehensive, expensive, and intensive measures – dietary alterations, exercise, statin and other drugs, and even coronary bypass surgeries and other procedures – are regularly undertaken to address plaque in arteries. Wouldn't it be great if doctors could learn a little about the associations between thyroid hormone replacement and the prevention of atherosclerosis? Of course! Sadly, even if the internist, cardiologist, or endocrinologist were aware of this association and dared to consider thyroid hormone to lower cholesterol and prevent plaque, they would either be severely limited or prevented entirely by the likely presence of a normal TSH, even in the very symptomatic patient with cholesterol levels in the 300s.

You see, a normal TSH always trumps abnormal clinical assessment findings because the TSH – a number – is considered to be more "evidence-based." In contrast, clinical assessment of the patient offers few numbers to report or track and is therefore not considered "evidence-based" in the eyes of many doctors. Findings are only valid as genuine "evidence" if they can be tested by a lab and reported as a number. (How convenient.) Therefore, because of the misleading TSH test – which usually hides the diagnosis of hypothyroidism – we no longer use thyroid to lower cholesterol in hypothyroid patients. Instead, our primary option is to rely on man-made pharmaceutical products explicitly designed to reduce cholesterol – and do *nothing* to address the underlying hormonal cause of elevated cholesterol. See how that works?

There's also a question about whether statins even inhibit the accumulation of plaque in the vessels as well as thyroid does. There's very little research on that particular issue – no surprise. I did find one head-to-head trial done in Istanbul, Turkey, in 2007, titled "Simvastatin improves endothelial function in patents [sic] with subclinical hypothyroidism."[5] In this study, the authors "compared the effects of simvastatin versus levothyroxine (LT-4) treatment on lipid profile and endothelial function in patients with SCH" (sub-clinical hypothyroidism). As the title suggests, the results showed significant benefits with the simvastatin and no significant benefit with thyroid hormone. However, they did admit that they found a trend that showed a benefit from thyroid, but it did not reach statistical significance.

Of course, the huge problem with this study was that a standard uniform dose of 100 mcg of T4 daily was given to all the thyroid patients, with no consideration of the level of clinical benefit. That small dose was likely inadequate for almost all patients; therefore, the lack of benefit isn't surprising. It's like giving 5 units of insulin to an entire group of diabetic patients, and when it doesn't adequately control their diabetes, concluding that insulin isn't a good diabetes treatment.

We've all been taught by the NIH, FDA, academic experts, and their friends in the drug industry that randomized, double-blind, placebo-controlled clinical trials yield the best data quality and are more "valid" than other types of medical studies. The primary problem with these studies is that, as seen in this case, the researchers give everyone a uniform dosage of the tested drug. This approach creates a tremendous bias against *any* therapy, including thyroid hormone replacement, where an effective dosage is carefully titrated to the individual patient's needs

Claiming that randomized trials are superior to other types of trials will *always* disadvantage drugs like thyroid hormone or insulin. Consequently, data derived from studies where thyroid hormone is clinically titrated to a unique dose in each patient will always be considered sub-par. It's a catch-22. Good thing that insulin hit the market before the FDA was created! Insulin probably wouldn't even be approved for use these days in the age of the precious randomized, double-blind, placebo-controlled trial!

Evaluating the effectiveness of thyroid hormone in preventing health issues and complications requires that we recognize that the hormone must be carefully titrated to obtain the optimal dose for each patient. But doing that takes time and a certain amount of clinical insight, and it sacrifices the nice, neat uniformity expected in today's drug company trials. Is it any surprise that I believe that randomized, double-blind, placebo-controlled trials will *never* reveal the actual benefits of thyroid replacement?

Suppose we want to measure the benefits of thyroid hormone replacement properly. In that case, we need to focus on clinical outcomes, like those presented in Broda Barnes' groundbreaking book, *Hypothyroidism, the Unsuspected Illness.*[6] His book is tremendously helpful and enlightening since he showed the results of doing thyroid replacement correctly, for example, diagnosing the condition clinically and giving enough thyroid to each patient to relieve the signs and symptoms present in that patient. He then compared the overall health outcomes of his patients managed in this manner to the outcomes of a similar group of controls from the Framingham data pool – patients who had not had their hypothyroidism (if present) diagnosed and managed in this manner. And his patients ended up simply healthier overall compared to the Framingham patients.

This is the best and most ethical way to measure outcomes when your goal is to prevent disease with a product that requires different doses for different patients. Rather than assessing the effects of a particular dose of thyroid hormone given to all the study subjects, Barnes evaluated the outcomes of using a *clinically titrated approach* to thyroid hormone replacement. Every hypothyroid patient is unique; therefore, they should receive a unique dose of thyroid replacement appropriate for their own individual needs. To think or do otherwise is a waste of time and a fool's errand.

CHAPTER 2: HOW TO DIAGNOSE HYPOTHYROIDISM: GENERAL PRINCIPLES

"Observe, record, tabulate, communicate. Use your five senses. Learn to see, learn to hear, learn to feel, learn to smell, and know that by practice alone you can become expert."
~ Sir William Osler

My medical training taught me that the foundation of a good diagnosis is a thorough medical history and physical exam, emphasizing the history part. This chapter reviews my beliefs about what should go into that history and exam.

THE VALUE OF A GOOD HISTORY AND AN OPEN MIND – ACCORDING TO OSLER AND OTHERS

Decades before the world of medicine was subject to the term "best practices" – a modern term that suggests that all patients should be treated the same and that there is one best way to treat all patients – Dr. Theodore Woodward, my professor of medicine at the University of Maryland School of Medicine back in the 1970s was teaching a very different approach. Dr. Woodward taught us that a good history and physical exam were crucial and that 85% of all diagnoses could be obtained from the history alone. (Dr.

Woodward must have known something about good health since he lived to the ripe old age of 92!)

During his lectures, he was fond of quoting Canadian physician Sir William Osler, a superb diagnostician considered to be the "Father of Modern Medicine." One of his favorite gems from Dr. Osler: "If you just listen to the patient, they will usually tell you what is wrong!" Dr. Osler was a founding professor of Johns Hopkins Hospital and created the first residency program for specialty training of physicians. Dr. Osler was also the first to expand medical training *beyond* lectures and into bedside clinical training. To this day, I am grateful and honored to have been taught medicine by a disciple of Sir William Osler.

I remember Dr. Woodward peering over his half glasses out at the eager students in the lecture hall in downtown Baltimore telling us in his soft but convincing voice, "If it looks, smells, and tastes like TB, it probably is!" That was his version of Osler's advice to "use your five senses, learn to see, learn to hear, learn to feel, learn to smell, and know that by practice alone you can become expert."

Osler also said, "He who studies medicine without books sails an uncharted sea, but he who studies medicine without patients, does not go to sea at all." In other words, patients provide valuable insights about their condition, and physicians should always pay attention to what patients are saying. Sadly, too many modern doctors never learned this crucial concept. Even if they did, they don't have the time to take advantage of this skill and instead rely only on lab tests, electronic algorithms, and checklists to make formulaic diagnoses.

Another of Sir William Osler's memorable quotes is the following: "Gentlemen, I have a confession to make. Half of what we have taught you is in error, and furthermore, we can't tell you which half it is." This, of course, suggests that we should always keep an open mind about what we have been taught because we are constantly learning new information about medicine. Sometimes we learn that what we thought was true is wrong. Therefore, we should all accept that "the science" is never "settled." In centuries past, doctors thought they could cure bad headaches by drilling holes in a patient's head! And not that long ago, we blamed stomach ulcers on "stress" and spicy foods and treated them with milk or antacids. Treatments should and do constantly evolve as we continue to learn. For example, we now know that ulcers are due to a bacterial infection in the stomach lining and that milk can make ulcers worse, so we now treat them with antibiotics instead of milk!

REPLACING CLINICAL ASSESSMENT WITH LAB TESTS HIDES THE DIAGNOSIS

Medical thinking has evolved over time, and while that's often a good thing, there *are* exceptions. Today's hypothyroidism care has wandered far from Osler's principles of patient-centered diagnosis, only to be replaced by reliance on lab tests. Absurdly, I have seen thyroid lecturers refer to the use of only lab tests as "evidence-based medicine." For them, a diagnosis based on TSH test results, excluding clinical findings and patient symptoms, is better "evidence" than a careful medical history and physical exam. And as for the validity of labs for the assessment of hypothyroidism, despite years of reading and asking endocrinologists, I have never found any data that prove that the TSH is a valid measurement of thyroid *function.* Yet "most experts agree" that TSH *measures thyroid function, despite the absence of* objective proof for that sacred belief.

Osler and Woodward would be turning over in their respective graves if they knew how "modern" medicine treats hypothyroidism.

That one misguided change in thyroid management – replacing careful clinical assessment of patients with total reliance on lab tests – is likely why you're reading this book.

FOCUS ON FUNCTION

If physicians are to improve the care of hypothyroid patients, we need to return to the principles of Sir William Osler and Dr. Theodore Woodward. We need to focus on thyroid *function.* Physicians must listen to what patients say when they explain what is wrong and trust what they say – even if the labs say something else. It's quite clear. Either the patients with all these clinical findings and symptoms are lying to us, or what we have been dogmatically taught to believe about lab tests is simply wrong. I'm quite confident it's the latter.

Thyroid tests measure thyroid hormone in the bloodstream, but they *don't* measure whether or not that thyroid hormone is actually working inside the cells. Tests count all the thyroid hormone, including the molecules that don't work.

An analogy I have used to explain this concept to my patients is to compare the bloodstream to a lazy river in a water park. Let's say that there are 100 inner tubes in the lazy river. But can 100 people float at the same time? Ask an endocrinologist, and they'll say "yes." They'll assume all the inner tubes are inflated and can support a rider. The careful clinician has a different take and would ask, "What proportion of those inner tubes are even inflated?" "Do some tubes have holes, and they're leaking air?" If only half the inner tubes are functional, then only 50 people can float. The mere presence of an inner tube in the lazy river – doesn't mean it's a functioning inner tube any more than the presence of thyroid hormone molecules in the bloodstream indicates functioning thyroid hormone. You need to look much more closely to actually measure function.

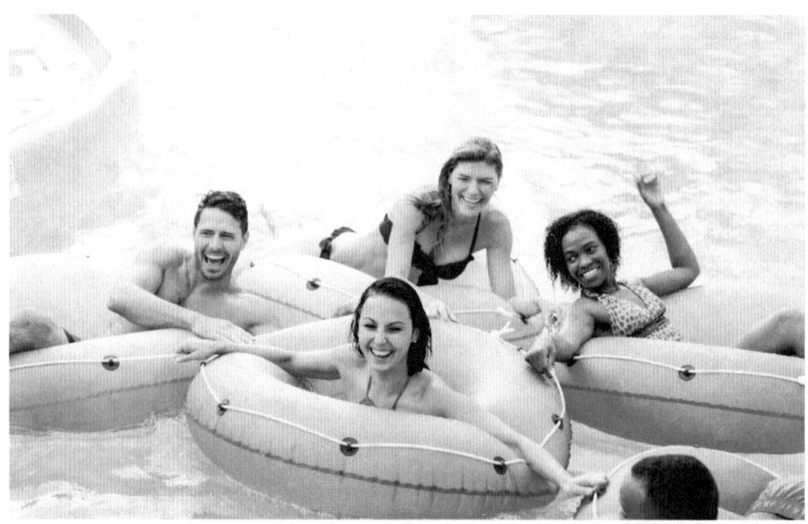

Since thyroid tests assume that all the thyroid hormones measured are fully functional, thyroid tests *overestimate* thyroid function. That's precisely why I believe lab tests are almost worthless for diagnosing hypothyroidism. Even so, thyroid antibodies tests, reverse T3, free T3, free T4, and thyroid sonograms can help obtain certain information about the thyroid gland. But *none* of these tests measure thyroid *function*. I wish the physicians, advocates, and hypothyroid self-help blogs and websites would spend less time recommending that patients get costly batteries of tests and instead encourage patients to identify doctors who are willing to focus more closely on careful clinical assessment.

TSH IS THEIR GOD!

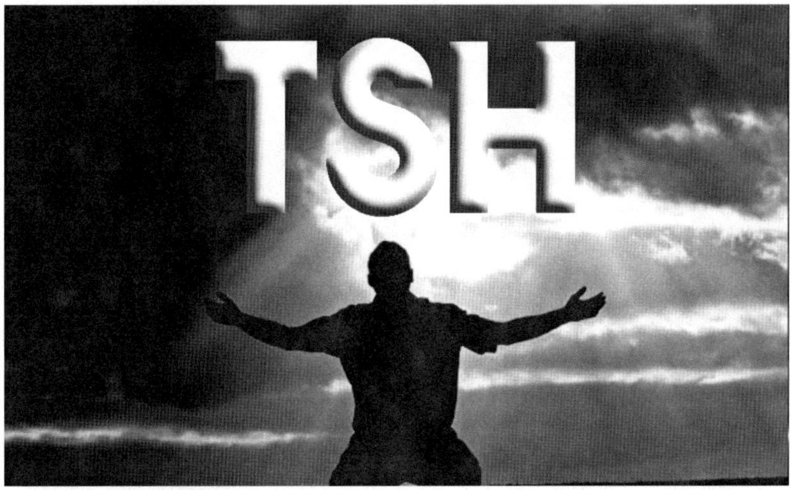

Many years ago, I had a patient, a nurse, who was quite difficult to manage. She was not following directions, not self-monitoring for symptoms of over- or under-medication, and, no surprise, she also wasn't getting well with my care. I encouraged her to seek care elsewhere since I could not help her, and her lack of following directions made me nervous. She saw an endocrinologist at good old Dr. Osler's Johns Hopkins Medical Center. (Note: the practice of medicine at Hopkins has changed quite a bit since Osler's time!) She was seen by the chairman of the Endocrinology Department, who was a prominent "thyroid expert."

After seeing her, he sent me a note carefully describing his findings, all of which suggested a diagnosis of *hypo*thyroidism and didn't support a diagnosis of *hyper*thyroidism. But because her TSH was suppressed on the dose she was taking, he diagnosed her as having "hypermedicamentosa," i.e., iatrogenic *hyper*thyroidism. In plain English, based entirely on the blood test results, he thought she had too *much* thyroid hormone, even though she had absolutely no clinical findings that would suggest that. Again, he was only thinking with his lab test results, not his eyes and ears. I then sent him a polite note asking him to explain why he decided she was *hyper*thyroid, even though none of his clinical findings supported that diagnosis. And I questioned his exclusive use of the TSH despite the conflicting physical findings. Specifically, I asked:

> *"Could you please offer some data which show that TSH actually measures all the multiple and complex functions of thyroid hormone? I understand it reflects the amount of thyroid hormone seen by the pituitary, but how does that measure intracellular function?"*

His response was the following:

> *"You know that the serum TSH is used to assess thyroid hormone levels, not only in the pituitary, but as a reflection of the hormonal status of the individual. I do not think that any additional discussion about this point would be fruitful."*[7]

No data or further explanation was offered. After all, how dare I question the validity of the sacrosanct TSH? I should know better. End of discussion. It's obvious that this attitude is widespread (though not quite universal) among the endocrinology community because, sadly, many of my patients have encountered this exact situation – but with less civility!

Osler was right. "The greater the ignorance, the greater the dogmatism!" Or, the more modern version, "Their ignorance is only exceeded by their arrogance."

PRE-VISIT SYMPTOM CHECKLIST

In my practice, the first step with a new thyroid patient was to have them fill out a pre-visit symptom checklist. I put together some of the most common – and telling – symptoms I encountered, and having patients fill out this form before our first appointment was informative and efficient.

I've included the form here, and please feel free to use this form yourself if you wish. My checklist isn't all-inclusive, but it gives a handy framework to collect enough data to know what is wrong with the patient so that you can aim your therapy in the right direction. There are many other versions of hypothyroidism symptoms lists all over the internet as well.

Donna Hurlock, MD

HYPOTHYROIDISM/LOW THYROID SYMPTOMS CHECKLIST

Name ______________________________ Date ______________

	Mild	Moderate	Severe
Fatigue	______	______	______
Weight gain	______	______	______
Depression	______	______	______
Anxiety	______	______	______
Memory Issues	______	______	______
Focus Issues (ADHD)	______	______	______
Migraines	______	______	______
Poor Sleep	______	______	______
Cold Intolerance	______	______	______
Heat Intolerance	______	______	______
Low Body Temperature	______	______	______
Hot Flashes	______	______	______
Cold Hands/Feet	______	______	______
Dry/Itchy Skin	______	______	______
Dry Eyes	______	______	______
Hair Loss	______	______	______
Water Retention	______	______	______
High Blood Pressure	______	______	______
Cravings	______	______	______
Constipation	______	______	______
High Cholesterol	______	______	______
Nasty Periods	______	______	______
Irregular Periods	______	______	______
Fertility Issues	______	______	______
No Sex Drive	______	______	______
Achy Joints	______	______	______
Achy Muscles	______	______	______
Tingling	______	______	______
Sensitive to Medicines	______	______	______
Sensitive to Coffee	______	______	______
______________	______	______	______
______________	______	______	______
______________	______	______	______

WHAT SYMPTOMS SHOULD I ASK ABOUT?

Sir William Osler said, "Variability is the law of life, and as no two faces are the same, so no two bodies are alike, and no two individuals react alike and behave alike under the abnormal conditions which we know as disease."

As Dr. Osler knew long ago, the first thing to know about the signs and symptoms of hypothyroidism is that all hypothyroid patients aren't alike. In my practice, some patients lumbered into my office, overweight, with achy joints, thin, wispy, prematurely gray hair, or even wearing a wig. They had swollen ankles, looked tired and sad, their faces were puffy, and they had bags under their eyes. They often wore more clothing than anyone else because they were chronically cold. Some brought a family member or friend to take notes because their focus and memory were so impaired that they would barely remember much of the visit.

But other patients bounced in, thin as a rail, with a big smile, and were quite talkative. You'd never suspect that they were hypothyroid until you ask them some questions and learn about their total lack of appetite, history of lifelong constipation, prior suicide attempt, ice cold hands, absent periods, compulsive exercise routines, need for Adderall to have any energy at all. Some rely on anti-anxiety drugs to achieve some semblance of focused brain function. Clearly, not all hypothyroid patients are the same.

In my practice, those initial observations and the Pre-Visit Symptoms Checklist served as a starting point for an in-depth conversation during the new patient visit. Then, we'd proceed to a discussion of their symptoms, both in the past and present. Sometimes, I even had to play the role of a detective to find out what was really happening with a patient. The goal is to find out the patient's key symptoms and challenges and use that information to develop an effective treatment plan that focuses on eliminating symptoms.

When "clinical wellness" – not "laboratory wellness" – is the goal, it takes much more than simply ordering a battery of lab tests. It requires knowledge, time, and energy for the physician to thoroughly evaluate the hypothyroid patient and her symptoms. It's more work for the physician, but it's crucial.

OPEN-ENDED QUESTIONS ARE BEST

I always found it best to start by asking a patient very open-ended questions, like:

- What problems are you having?
- Which symptoms bother you the most?
- When did your symptoms begin?
- How long have your symptoms been present?
- When were you last feeling perfectly well?
- How severe and disabling are your symptoms?
- How have your symptoms changed over time?
- Are you able to function day-to-day with normal activities?
- Are you able to work and meet your family obligations?
- Did a particular event precede the onset of the symptoms? (Hypothyroidism symptoms can begin after mononucleosis, a whiplash neck injury, recent pregnancy, traumatic event, exposure to environmental radiation (such as the nuclear reactor incident in Chernobyl in 1986), or head and neck radiation treatment (commonly used in the 1970s to treat acne).

Most of the time, the symptoms identified at the first visit were significant enough to merit an immediate trial of thyroid replacement. But sometimes, if the patient had very mild symptoms like cold hands or feet but was otherwise functioning perfectly well, had a favorable cholesterol, and nothing threatened her well-being, we would decide that she didn't need treatment. That was particularly true in adolescent or teen patients since compliance is challenging in that age group. At the same time, I also knew that symptoms rarely improve on their own and often worsen over time. That's why I always left the door open to continue monitoring the patient so that we could begin treatment down the road.

However, if the patient had high cholesterol, I usually recommended starting treatment immediately since cholesterol almost always normalizes with proper thyroid replacement and fixing high cholesterol with thyroid is better than not fixing it or going straight to statin drugs!

LOOK FOR SIGNS OF SLUGGISH BODY FUNCTIONS

Remember that thyroid hormone acts as the accelerator pedal for all of our body processes. And, when there's too little pressure on our accelerator pedal, all our body functions become sluggish. Therefore, I would then move on to identify some of the common signs of sluggish body functions with more specific questions, such as:

- How much did you weigh when the symptoms started?
- Do you eat more or less than other people?
- Do you get full easily but want to nibble all day long?
- Do you need to eat a lot of food to get full at meals, or do tiny meals make you full?
- How much do you exercise?
- How much sleep do you get? How much sleep do you need to feel refreshed?
- Do you usually have a low temperature?
- Do your skin wounds heal slowly?
- Are you particularly sensitive to medications? Do you commonly take only part of your dose because you know a full dose will be too strong?
- Are you now less tolerant of coffee or alcohol than you were in the past?
- How is your mood? Do you feel depressed, anxious, or exhausted? How often?

Then I would ask about prior attempts to address these symptoms:

- Has anyone ever done thyroid lab tests?

- Do you have the most current values with you?
- Has anyone ever treated you for a thyroid condition in the past?
- What thyroid medicines have you tried in the past, at what doses, and what was your response to those doses?
- Have you ever seen an endocrinologist? How many?
- Has their treatment helped you? (Hint: If it had, they would likely not have been sitting in my office!)

PERSONAL AND FAMILY HISTORY ARE IMPORTANT

Many factors are especially important to include when taking a history of a potentially hypothyroid patient. These include:

- Personal or family history of any thyroid condition or exposure to any thyrotoxin like radiation, environmental chemicals, chemotherapy, or even neck trauma
- Residing in an area where dietary iodine is deficient, a "goiter belt"
- Personal or family history of autoimmune disease
- Other past or current diagnoses
- Past surgeries
- Pregnancy history
- Onset of menstruation
- Onset of menopause
- Current medications
- Current supplements
- Any allergies

WHAT CAUSES HYPOTHYROIDISM – GENES OR THE ENVIRONMENT?

It's very common for hypothyroid patients to have family members who are also hypothyroid. Therefore, you can rightly say that it can "run in families," but I don't believe hypothyroidism is primarily transmitted genetically in most cases. Instead, I suspect it has more to do with common environmental exposures.

I always asked about thyroid disease in the family because having a first-degree relative with a thyroid condition – a parent, sibling, or child – puts a woman at higher risk for a thyroid condition. We also live in a veritable soup of environmental chemical compounds and radiation sources that are toxic to our thyroid glands. Sadly, families who live together often develop thyroid dysfunction due to common toxic exposures.

In his 2005 book, *Hypothyroidism Type 2*,[8] Mark Starr, MD, noted that almost 70,000 new synthetic compounds were introduced in the 20th century. Many of those are known to be thyrotoxins. He even included a list of hundreds of specific compounds known to be toxic to our thyroid glands. For example, PBDEs (polybrominated diphenyl esters) – the fire-retardant-chemicals used in mattresses and baby pajamas until they were banned in 2004 – are known as thyrotoxins. Now manufacturers are using OPFRs (organophosphate flame retardants) instead, and of course, we still don't have enough data on those to say they are safe.[9] Great, right? Sadly, most man-made chemical compounds have never even been tested to see if they have a potential for hormone toxicity. As a result, we usually don't find out about toxicity until after they have been in widespread use for years and the damage is done.

It turns out, for example, that many pesticides fall into the category of hormone disruptors, so a history of pesticide exposure should be evaluated. Hormone disruptors can interfere with many mammalian hormones, including estrogen, testosterone, and of course, thyroid. (The dramatic increase in exposure to hormone disruptors may also shed some light on the recent upswing in problems with both male and female infertility and problems with libido, among others.)

It's virtually impossible in our lifetimes to avoid exposing ourselves to some situations or substances that can damage our delicate thyroid glands. These types of exposures are frequently shared in families located in the same geographic area for extended periods. This is why I ask about where people grew up geographically. People who grew up in "goiter belts" – iodine-deficient regions like the American Great Lakes or the Alps in Europe – have a higher risk of thyroid problems. And people who lived downwind from nuclear reactors or in the area of nuclear accidents have an increased risk of many different thyroid conditions. I was taking a history on one new patient and learned that she had grown up in Russia and was living near Chernobyl when the nuclear reactor accident occurred in 1986. Knowing that, it was clear that her thyroid didn't stand a chance of remaining normal after that radiation exposure, and she also needed to be monitored for thyroid cancer.

EVEN ANIMALS HAVE THYROID DISEASE

America's Great Lakes are known to be polluted with many chemical contaminants. And it's no coincidence that both Coho and chinook salmon found in the Great Lakes have been found to have "thyroid hyperplasia and goiters, which appeared to have an environmental etiology. Researchers found[10] 13-fold differences in goiter prevalence within the Great Lakes."

In addition, according to the British Thyroid Foundation's website[11] and several of my veterinarian patients, thyroid disease is quite common in dogs, particularly Golden Retrievers and Dobermann Pinschers, and cats. Dogs tend to develop low thyroid function, and cats tend to become hyperthyroid. The British Thyroid Foundation states, "Hyperthyroidism in cats was first described in 1979 and is now the most common endocrine disorder. Risk factors have not been fully established but may be linked to chronic exposure to thyroid-disrupting chemicals in the environment."

For example, my two now-deceased cats, Ginger and Dollface, were both hyperthyroid. I know now that there is some evidence that the plastic coating that lines cat food cans can leach into the canned food and act as a hormone disruptor. Ginger was amenable to taking thyroid-blocking pills to treat it, and she lived until she was 18. But at age 11 and a weight of 4.5 pounds, Dollface refused to take any medication, spitting out her pills onto the floor and under furniture. As a result, she received radioactive iodine treatment to kill off her overactive thyroid gland.

After that very effective treatment, Dollface became hypothyroid, and my newly hypothyroid little kitty managed to live another 10 years to the age of 21! She gained some weight, shed lots of hair, slept a lot, and showed a consistent fondness for napping in sunny, warm spots in the house.

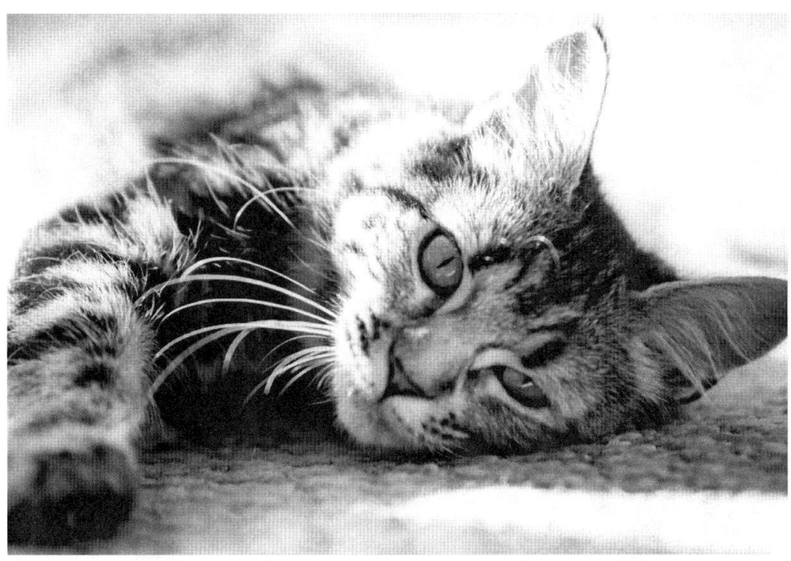

CLINICAL SIGNS OF HYPOTHYROIDISM: THE PHYSICAL EXAM

Before I discuss what goes into a complete physical exam for hypothyroidism, I want to raise an important point. The modern "physical" – which typically involves checking weight, blood pressure, and ordering a battery of lab tests for cholesterol, blood sugar, etc. – does NOT necessarily include *any* thyroid tests. More shockingly, the history is often very superficial and appears in the form of a check-off list on an iPad. There is minimal space for writing details or adding things not already on the list. Sometimes a physical exam is not even performed. This, of course, has gotten worse in the new age of telemedicine. (Countless patients of mine said I was the first doctor ever to do a hands-on exam, feeling their pulse, checking for thyroid enlargement, feeling skin texture, noticing ankle or facial swelling, and checking to see if the hands and feet are icy to the touch).

The provider or physician extender often misses all those physical clues as they focus on ordering dozens of lab tests to find the diagnosis. Due to this overreliance on blood tests and disagreement on how they're interpreted, patients are often told "your thyroid is fine," or they're left to a self-service process of retrieving their lab results from a portal and then going online to try to figure out what those results might mean. The concept of the "art of medicine" is long gone!

But if the physician truly wants to find the underlying cause of the patient's symptoms, then the old-fashioned art of careful observation must be revisited. Below are some things that need to be observed by the careful physician in any patient suspected to be hypothyroid.

- Measure weight and height. (Height is helpful when watching for osteoporosis).
- Check blood pressure.
- Pulse rate. Is it slow, irregular in any way, or weak? Are there any missed or extra beats?
- Hands-on external palpation of the thyroid gland to feel for any enlargement, lumps, bumps, or irregularities.
- Check reflexes. Do they appear sluggish or absent?
- Examine the hair for dryness or signs of thinning, shedding, receding, and premature graying.
- Examine the eyebrows for signs of thinning or loss of the outer third (a classic sign of hypothyroidism).

- Examine the nails, looking for vertical ridges, weakness, peeling, and breakage. Fungal infections of the toenails are suggestive.
- Look for swelling around the eyes, face, or tongue (scalloped edges).
- Look for swelling in the hands, feet, ankles, legs, and marks from socks or shoes.
- Evaluate hands and feet for coldness. The nose can often be cold as well.
- Evaluate the skin for dryness, eczema, psoriasis, vitiligo, rashes, slow healing of scratches, etc. (Thinness and wrinkling can suggest estrogen deficiency).
- Evaluate the feet for excessive calluses.
- Listen to the voice for hoarseness, deepness, or slowness of speech.
- Notice what the patient is wearing. Is it appropriate to the surrounding temperature?
- Is the patient's gait slow or sluggish?
- Does the patient appear focused? Is she slow to respond to questions? Is she having difficulty finding words? Did she bring someone with her to take notes, etc.?
- Are the patient's emotions normal, or is the patient's affect flat? Is she anxious or hyper?
- Is the patient yawning? Does she appear tired?

HYPOTHYROIDISM IS EXTREMELY COMMON

As you can see, with a discussion of symptoms, a detailed history, and a physical examination, a thorough and accurate diagnosis requires a new patient visit that is much longer than the typical "7 to 10-minute dash" that is the average for many doctor's visits in the U.S. That's why most of the doctors who approach thyroid the way I did don't accept the time limitations that are required by insurance plan participation.

But taking that time is essential.

When we use clinical assessment as a basis for a diagnosis, thyroid dysfunction is, frankly, *extremely* common. When you look closely and know what to look for, it seems that most of our thyroid glands become damaged at one time or another. Indeed, you can often find mothers and daughters, sisters, co-workers, etc., who all have hypothyroidism. In my case, not only am I hypothyroid, but so is my daughter, my late husband, my ex-husband, and his second ex-wife. And, of course, we can also include my cats, Dollface and Ginger.

Retrospectively, my dad was likely hypothyroid back in the 1960s, but he was never diagnosed. Instead, when my father was too tired, achy, and weak to go to work for an entire year, his young and modern doctor – straight out of his training at Johns Hopkins – diagnosed him with a condition called "Epidemic Neuromyasthenia" (That term literally means "we're seeing a lot of patients lately who are tired and achy and weak.") Not only was my dad too tired to work, but I remember that he always wore a sweatshirt to bed and had icy cold feet.

The TSH had just been introduced at that time, and clearly, my dad's doctor was an early believer in the superiority of that modern laboratory test. Since my dad's TSH was surely "in the normal range," his doctor had to come up with a new diagnosis other than hypothyroidism, which is why he was diagnosed with this mysterious new "epidemic" disease. The current day term for his ailment would be chronic fatigue syndrome or fibromyalgia.

Regrettably, if my dad had simply chosen an older doctor with a bit more experience under his belt, he would likely have been treated with thyroid and quickly recovered. Instead, the modern doctor's "care" caused him to spend a year at home, not working. Luckily, I was sheltered from the financial and emotional fallout of his extended illness. Still, it's part of the reason why I am so motivated to help people with hypothyroidism get their lives back.

PART 2: CLINICAL FINDINGS AND SYMPTOMS

CHAPTER 3: THE ROLE OF ESTROGEN

"It's time to stop grouping up and complaining about all our estrogen deficient symptoms and demand real answers and plenty of estrogen."
~ Marie Hoag

You may find it a bit odd that I'm starting this section of the book on diagnosis and management of hypothyroidism with a discussion of…estrogen. Why estrogen?

First, as a practicing gynecologist for decades, the women I treated rarely came to see me with just one specific hormonal issue. Most have been in their mid-life years and thus are affected by changing estrogen levels and thyroid dysfunction. The endocrine system is just that, a *system*, and hormones are highly interrelated and dependent on each other in many ways. Hormones like estrogen and progesterone, thyroid hormone, adrenal hormone, and insulin rarely "stay in their own lanes." They interact with and affect each other constantly throughout our lives. Some of their functions often overlap. And nowhere is that more evident than in the relationship between estrogen and thyroid hormone, especially in women in perimenopause and beyond.

Thus, to be successful in treating hypothyroidism, we also need to understand just what estrogen and estrogen deficiency do in our menopausal patients since many of those effects can mimic some of the effects of hypothyroidism. Further, the presence or absence or any change in the amount of estrogen present will affect thyroid function through resultant changes in sex hormone binding globulins (proteins) that are stimulated by estrogen. These binding globulins, in turn, affect reproductive hormones – but also affect thyroid hormone.

Consequently, when we start or stop estrogen therapy, we can also affect thyroid function. Specifically, stopping – or reducing – estrogen can enhance the effects of thyroid. Adding estrogen seems to blunt the effect of thyroid slightly. This is particularly true with patients who go on and off of birth control pills. But it can also be seen in women on hormone replacement who chose to go on and off of it. When they stop their estrogen, thyroid function increases slightly, and when they begin taking estrogen, thyroid function becomes a bit blunted.

Yet, to make things even more complicated, sometimes the reverse is true! On many occasions, I have seen a woman suddenly become hypothyroid shortly after experiencing natural or surgical menopause. It seems that perhaps the thyroid and the ovaries are best friends, and when the ovaries eventually fail, the thyroid goes into mourning and slows down its function. I don't exactly understand this and can't fully explain it, but it does seem to happen from time to time. You may want to read some of Mary Shomon's excellent books to learn more about this phenomenon.

But first, let's discuss some of the effects of estrogen on parts of the body that are also affected by thyroid hormone.

ESTROGEN AND THYROID DEFICIENCIES BOTH CAUSE VASOSPASMS AND VASOMOTOR SYMPTOMS

First, let's start by reviewing a few more basics about estrogen. You should know that our blood vessels are lined with estrogen and thyroid receptors, which are affected by the presence of both hormones in the bloodstream. Both estrogen and thyroid have two functions in the blood vessels. First, they act as vasodilators, keeping the vessels relaxed and open. Second, they keep the endothelial cells healthy and free of plaque. The blood vessels in the brain and the heart are especially rich in estrogen receptors.

We know from many human and animal studies that the sudden removal of estrogen – or significant fluctuations in estrogen levels – can cause something called a vasospasm. The term vasospasm refers to a contraction in the muscular walls of a blood vessel that causes it to narrow. This narrowing reduces the blood flow within that vessel. This can cause symptoms like hot flashes, which are "vasomotor symptoms."

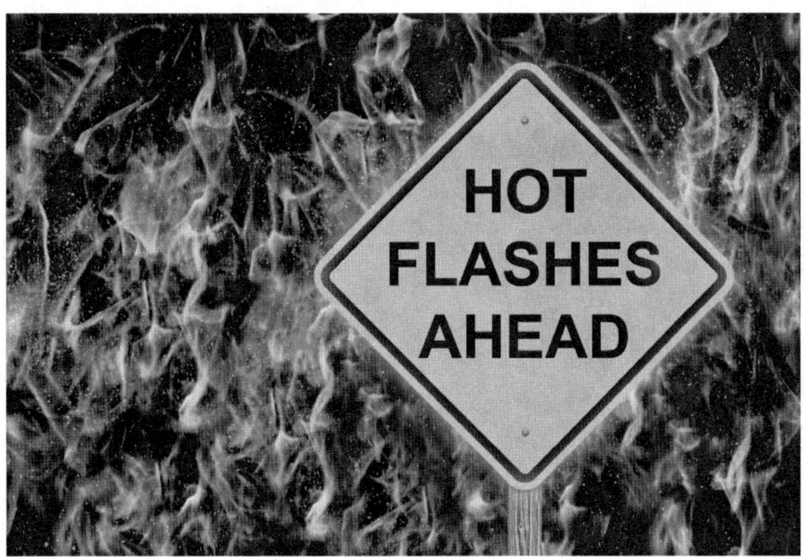

During a woman's reproductive years, she typically produces enough estrogen to keep her blood vessels happy and relaxed. However, there is one time during the menstrual cycle when there's a sudden, significant, natural drop in estrogen: right before the start of menstruation. The most common premenstrual vasomotor symptom is migraine, but some young women also report hot flashes.

During perimenopause in hypothyroid patients – which is defined as the phase before the cessation of menstrual periods – estrogen levels can fluctuate wildly, leading to more intense vasospasms and symptoms. In some women, these fluctuations can start as early as their late 30s, and this phase can continue for up to a decade until estrogen levels finally drop to such a low point that menstrual periods stop entirely. During this time of hormonal fluctuation, the most common vasomotor symptoms should be familiar: hot flashes and night sweats.

When a woman hasn't menstruated for one year, she is labeled as officially menopausal, and from that point onward, she is considered postmenopausal.

When a woman is postmenopausal – even when she's not on hormone replacement therapy – her vasospasms and resulting vasomotor symptoms usually go away slowly over time. After being deprived of estrogen for a long time, estrogen receptors in the vessel walls finally enter a dormant stage and can no longer respond to the lack of estrogen. The receptors essentially get tired of waiting for an estrogen molecule to float by, so they go "off the clock."

Why am I telling you this in a discussion of thyroid? Because estrogen is highly sensitive to thyroid levels, hypothyroid women tend to have more intense responses to sudden drops and fluctuations in estrogen levels and more exaggerated peaks and valleys in estrogen levels due to slowed estrogen clearance by the sluggish hypothyroid liver. Women with hypothyroidism also commonly report more migraines and more temperature dysregulation.

I understand that this is a bit complicated. Still, the bottom line is this: any sudden drop in estrogen levels can create vasospasms and vasomotor symptoms like migraines, hot flashes, and night sweats. Further, these symptoms can also occur due to hypothyroidism. And when these symptoms occur due to hypothyroidism, they are often misdiagnosed as being due to menopause, even though the patient still has plenty of estrogen. Before I learned much about hypothyroidism, I used to think that all hot flashes were due to dropping estrogen levels, but I now know that is far from the truth. Because thyroid function affects estrogen levels, and vice versa, resolving these symptoms requires careful management of *both* the thyroid *and* the estrogen levels. When a woman has vasomotor symptoms, we need to look at optimizing thyroid function – *and* estrogen levels as well.

Due to their fear of estrogen, some menopausal women try to just replace just thyroid and not replace estrogen. Unfortunately, just replacing one of these hormones without the other never works. If both hormones are deficient, both need to be adequately replaced to resolve these vasomotor symptoms. There are two reasons for this.

1. If you replace thyroid and do not replace estrogen, the added thyroid will make the estrogen deficiency worse
2. If you give only estrogen and not thyroid hormone, the estrogen will block the woman's thyroid function, which is already inadequate.

The two hormones are, in a sense, fighting each other. But the bottom line is this: If you want to fix symptoms due to vasospasms, both hormones need to be replaced simultaneously. I learned this the hard way by trying the "one hormone" approach on several patients. I would not recommend that practitioners or patients waste time trying that approach!

Why is it that estrogen and thyroid seem to fight each other? When a menopausal woman isn't taking adequate estrogen, adding thyroid hormone reduces estrogen levels. The thyroid revs up the liver, getting it to start conjugating the small amount of estrogen in a postmenopausal woman's bloodstream. She ends up metabolizing away some of her already scarce estrogen at the same time. The unintended consequence is that all sorts of estrogen deficiency symptoms can recur.

For example, suppose thyroid hormone replacement is started in a 60-year-old menopausal woman who isn't on estrogen replacement and who hasn't had any hot flashes for at least five years. Shortly after starting a dose of thyroid, her hot flashes return. Those hot flashes are likely due to worsening estrogen deficiency – *not* due to thyroid overdose. In addition, the reduction in estrogen level caused by increasing the metabolism (also known as the "clearance") of her estrogen will almost always worsen the quality of her sleep. As a result, now that she has started thyroid – which is telling her liver to chew up her estrogen faster – she is also waking up with night sweats. Trust me when I say that most women will *not* be pleased with this outcome. So please replace both if both are missing!

ESTROGEN AND THYROID DEFICIENCIES BOTH DISRUPT SLEEP

Like hot flashes and night sweats, sleep problems are common in both hypothyroid and estrogen-deficient women. Studies have shown that the human brain is filled with estrogen and thyroid hormone receptors. The brain can't perform well, and women will experience ongoing sleep disruptions – not to mention fatigue and brain fog – when there's inadequate estrogen or thyroid hormone.

This is particularly problematic in perimenopause and early menopause when the blood vessels are still relatively supple and capable of significant vasospasms. What happens in these women is that their estrogen deficiency causes the blood vessels to spasm episodically, which, in turn, causes hot flashes or night sweats, which then awakens a woman in the middle of the night with a soaked nightgown and sheets.

Many sleep-deprived hypothyroid patients are also estrogen deficient, so never ignore the effects of menopause. Just as replacing thyroid hormone is the best way to control symptoms caused by thyroid deficiency, the best way to manage symptoms caused by estrogen deficiency, such as hot flashes, night sweats, and sleep disruption, is to replace estrogen. That's why I started postmenopausal hypothyroid patients who wanted to sleep well on both thyroid hormone replacement *and* estrogen replacement – *at the same time.* The two hormones work together to improve sleep quality and other neurologic functions and I had much greater success replacing both rather than just replacing thyroid.

If a woman has become menopausal fairly recently, no problem! It's safe and easy to do both. The *only* exception to this approach is when a patient already has a significant amount of plaque in her arteries, which makes initiating estrogen therapy hazardous. In these cases, I explained the situation to my patient. We then aimed to get as much benefit as possible with thyroid treatment without exacerbating any symptoms of estrogen deficiency, such as poor sleep, sweats, hot flashes, or bone loss.

PLAQUE IS NOT A PATIENT'S FRIEND: HOW AND WHEN TO ASSESS PLAQUE BURDEN

As soon as a woman hits menopause, plaque – hardening of the arteries and atherosclerosis – begins accumulating in the vessel walls.[12] This plaque accumulates slowly over time, making the vessels gradually more rigid. When receptors are covered with plaque and relatively rigid, the vessels can no longer sense estrogen deficiency and vasospasms typically stop. In one sense, that's good because the hot flashes and night sweats are gone, and women may have fewer sleep problems. At the same time, it suggests that the vessels have deteriorated and are becoming atherosclerotic, and that's never good.

Hodis demonstrated in his EPAT trial in 2001[13] that statistically significant amounts of plaque will accumulate in the vessels of a woman in early menopause within just 2 years of living without estrogen. This alone is a compelling reason always to begin replacing estrogen as soon as it becomes deficient. Interestingly, according to Broda Barnes' 1976 book, *The Riddle of Heart Attacks*,[14] a similar situation occurs with prolonged thyroid deficiency.

If a woman has been postmenopausal for a long time and has developed significant plaque during that timeframe, it's no longer safe to begin estrogen because we know that estrogen destabilizes existing plaque and can cause emboli. If estrogen sees plaque, it breaks it into little pieces that can float down the bloodstream and cause serious problems like strokes and heart attacks. That's why it's crucial to begin hormone replacement at the onset of menopause, long before any plaque can accumulate. If you don't have significant plaque, estrogen will not cause any of these problems and will only protect your blood vessels.

Before considering estrogen or thyroid replacement, I always assessed whether my postmenopausal patients had significant levels of pre-existing plaque in their arteries. While no standard "expert guidelines" address this fundamental issue, here's how I handled it.

First, I asked the patient if she had any history of heart disease or had ever had her blood vessels imaged. Has she ever seen a cardiologist? If there had been no issues, and if the patient had been estrogen deficient for less than 10 years and had no unusual risk factors for plaque, such as a history of heavy smoking, I assumed her blood vessels were still clean, and I proceeded with initiating HRT. This assumption is based on the Women's Health Initiative data showing a decrease in mortality in estrogen users who were under the age of 60 at the start of the study.[15] The fact that there was a *decrease* in mortality would suggest that the vessels were clear of plaque. If not, there perhaps would have been a slight increase in mortality, as they saw in the WHI in the women over the age of 70 at the onset of the study, most of whom likely had some significant plaque.

On the other hand, if the patient were estrogen deficient for more than ten years or had any other risk factors for plaque, I would proceed to the next step: getting a coronary calcium score. Since a coronary calcium score is a CT scan of the heart, and there is a bit of radiation involved, I don't recommend doing this test yearly. It is, however, more sensitive than a carotid doppler and safer and less invasive than an angiogram. This test counts flecks of calcium seen along the course of the coronary arteries. If the score is 0, meaning no calcified plaque is seen, my patient and I would celebrate, and she would immediately begin supplemental estrogen.

If the score was above 0 but was low, for example, less than 40 to 50, I discussed the results with my patient, and we reviewed how the benefits of beginning estrogen replacement outweighed the risks. If the value was higher, I generally shied away from beginning HRT. Instead, I referred that patient to a cardiologist for a second opinion and possible management of her risk factors.

It would be nice if there were some evidence-based guidelines to help us decide the best cut-off value, but sadly, we don't have such data at this time, and I'm not sure we ever will. However, a couple of years ago, I did discuss this protocol with Howard Hodis, MD, who is, in my opinion, the guru of studying the effect of estrogen on blood vessels. Dr. Hodis thought it was very reasonable and prudent.

In general, while brief periods without estrogen are fine, if a woman of average risk has been without estrogen for 10 years or more, we should assume that she has developed moderate plaque and only consider replacing estrogen in that patient if a vascular study like a coronary calcium score demonstrates that the vessels are relatively clean. Happily, in many patients, that was the case, and they safely began replacing estrogen. However, those patients with moderate or severe levels of plaque in their vessels (because they missed the HRT "window of opportunity") needed to avoid estrogen replacement and focus on thyroid replacement.

ESTROGEN DEFICIENCY TRIGGERS MIGRAINE HEADACHES

I discuss migraine in greater depth in Chapter 12, but I mention it here because migraine is so often related to estrogen levels. Honestly, the ability to cure chronic migraine headaches is often one of the easiest and most rewarding results of replacing thyroid properly. Chronic migraines are tremendously debilitating, and current standard treatments involve expensive and side-effect-laden medicines and procedures like Botox injections that, in too many cases, offer limited control of the problem. To completely cure a patient's tendency to have migraine headaches is a godsend, and I am very grateful to have been able to do this for my migraine patients on a fairly regular basis.

To fix migraines, it's crucial that a patient has adequate estrogen throughout the month and that fluctuations are minimized. In menopausal women, I would usually use continuous estrogen patches since they yield an even serum level throughout the month with smaller daily fluctuations than those you get with oral estrogen. In women still menstruating, I recommend a 0.1 mg estrogen patch during the few days before and immediately after the onset of the period when estrogen drops to its lowest level. If replacing and smoothing out estrogen fluctuations is inadequate and a patient is hypothyroid, I suggest adding T4 to achieve an increased metabolic rate and heat production. It works better than T3 for increasing heat production and opening peripheral and cranial blood vessels. Once a patient is on enough thyroid to make the hands and feet consistently warm, the headaches are usually gone. It's life-changing!

TREATING WITH ESTROGEN

I want to recap a critical point that practitioners and patients need to understand. When an estrogen-deficient woman is treated with thyroid hormone, her estrogen deficiency will become more pronounced, manifesting as an increase in menopausal symptoms. Thyroid hormone isn't directly causing hot flashes, migraine, or sleep disturbances. Instead, when a woman has very little estrogen in her bloodstream, to begin with, the addition of thyroid hormone increases the clearance rate of estrogen, making the estrogen level go so low that symptoms of estrogen deficiency can recur.

When this happens, what is the best way to resolve this problem? Without fail, the natural inclination of women and many doctors will be to stop or reduce the thyroid medication, thinking that the thyroid dose is too high. But the correct answer is to begin treating the estrogen deficiency with estrogen.

I know that some women are reluctant to take estrogen because they've heard from friends and Dr. Google that estrogen immediately turns into a cardiotoxic carcinogen the minute you hit 50. But I'm here to dispel that myth. All hormones interact with each other, and patients will never achieve optimal wellness with thyroid if estrogen remains deficient.

Assuming that blood vessels are still relatively free of plaque, full estrogen "hormone" replacement is the only treatment that is going to work, preferably using a non-oral product like the patch or one of the topical gels so that the serum estrogen level remains relatively constant throughout the day and night.

If estrogen levels are tested, the target should be a moderate level well above the normal menopausal range. I never liked wasting health care dollars by ordering unnecessary and misleading lab tests, so I usually relied on clinical clues to determine whether or not the dose was adequate. Specifically, I tried to give enough estrogen to make the patient's breasts "awake" but not painful. By "awake," I mean that the breasts feel slightly sensitive, like when the patient had periods. That way, when I added in thyroid medication, the estrogen dropped somewhat, but not so low that all those symptoms of estrogen deficiency and menopause appeared. The dose of estrogen that keeps the breasts "awake" will also protect bones, blood vessels, and the brain.

Living without estrogen for many years after menopause is a recipe for developing an increasingly problematic burden of plaque. I don't recommend it, and those physicians who advise their patients to avoid estrogen replacement completely are misinformed and bordering on malpractice, in my opinion. A book published in 2018 titled *Estrogen Matters*,[16] written by retired oncologist Avrum Bluming, MD, and psychologist Carol Tavris, Ph.D., is an excellent source of information and references. This book effectively explains why estrogen replacement is crucial if one wants to preserve a woman's good health after menopause. This even applies to breast cancer survivors. I encourage all menopausal women and the physicians who care for them to read that book. (I wish I had written it!)

To be clear, it's almost always safe and advisable to start HRT early in menopause and continue it until death. In fact, I highly recommend it and am doing that myself. The one caveat: women shouldn't start HRT well after the onset of menopause unless it's first proven that they don't have significant plaque, because then, the estrogen can create a shower of micro emboli. As mentioned earlier, my routine for this was to do a cardiac calcium score if the patient had been without estrogen for 10 years or more before starting HRT. I would also evaluate for plaque before initiating estrogen replacement if the particular patient had significant risk factors for plaque, like a long history of smoking or prior vascular issues. If there is little or no plaque, that's a green light to start HRT. But in the presence of significant plaque, even I did not prescribe HRT. Instead, I referred patients to a cardiologist to manage modifiable risk factors.

In conclusion, from the thyroid perspective, if you want to completely resolve symptoms like migraines, hot flashes, night sweats, poor sleep, and brain fog, menopausal patients will enjoy far more successful treatment when they're concurrently on full-dose HRT.

BUT WHAT ABOUT ESTROGEN AND BREAST CANCER?

Since we are talking about estrogen replacement and contraindications to estrogen, we need to also touch on the widespread misconception that estrogen replacement makes breast cancer worse or that it somehow causes breast cancer. I suspect that most women and their physicians currently believe that estrogen and breast cancer are related. I was certainly told that during my Ob-Gyn residency in the early 1980s! I was cautioned that "you should never prescribe estrogen replacement to a breast cancer patient." Of course, I believed it back then because it made sense. Estrogen "fed" cancer; therefore, it surely made cancer worse.

The problem is that the data show *just the opposite.* Yes, estrogen feeds estrogen receptor-positive breast cancer cells, but estrogen also feeds normal breast cells, bone cells, and brain cells, among other cells. All of these cells have estrogen receptors, meaning estrogen is expected to attach to them to stimulate those cells.

Estrogen is indeed a trophic hormone, meaning it makes things grow, but that alone does not mean that cancer outcomes are worse in the presence of estrogen or that estrogen is a carcinogen. To determine that, one needs to look at the clinical data instead of just dwelling on theoretical concepts like the presence or absence of estrogen receptors.

We could start by noticing that after many woman-year studies of oral contraceptives, the body of literature fails to show a positive relationship between the use of birth control pills and breast cancer. And we should remember that an average low-dose birth control pill contains about four to six times the amount of estrogen found in a typical day's dose of HRT. The FDA and others want us to believe that a supraphysiologic dose of estrogen – like in birth control pills – does *not* cause breast cancer, but a smaller replacement dose, such as in HRT, does. Does that make sense? No.

Further, breast cancer isn't more common in young women of reproductive age who have high estrogen levels. Instead, it's most commonly found in the very elderly, who have almost no estrogen. The association of breast cancer incidence with age is positive and very linear, occurring more commonly as one gets older, and is inversely related to the times when women have the most estrogen.

Indeed, the clinical evidence that we have on the relationship between HRT and breast cancer shows that women who are on HRT at the time they are diagnosed with breast cancer have a much *higher* survival rate than women who are diagnosed with breast cancer when they aren't on HRT. Breast cancers found in estrogen users tend to be smaller, more confined, and of a less aggressive grade than those found in women who aren't on estrogen. In reality, HRT seems to work like mammography; as a diagnostic aide, it helps expose cancers at an earlier stage. And guess what? If you find breast cancer at an early stage, it's easier to cure.

Further, contrary to popular belief, women who continue on their HRT *after* their diagnosis of breast cancer *do not* have increased recurrence rates. Additionally, they have about a 40% reduction in all-cause mortality compared to those obedient breast cancer patients who take the advice of their oncologists and stop their HRT at the time of diagnosis.[17] Would I stop my estrogen if I were diagnosed with breast cancer? Absolutely not.

It is also interesting to note that back in the 1970s, the package insert for Premarin included an FDA-approved indication for the palliative treatment of advanced breast cancer. In fact, a 2016 study from the Netherlands, "The use of high-dose estrogens for the treatment of breast cancer," suggests that it's "an effective treatment for this disease" and it "should be considered a valuable alternative to chemotherapy in selected patients."[18]

While the literature shows the benefits of *treating* breast cancer with estrogen, the current package inserts for all estrogens – including vaginally applied estrogen creams – list breast cancer as a contraindication. It's unclear why that indication for palliative treatment of advanced breast cancer was quietly removed from the package insert and replaced with a black box warning. (It might have something to do with the FDA's relationship with the drug industry and their lack of enthusiasm for effective and relatively inexpensive measures that can prevent disease, such as hormone replacement therapy. If you detect a trend here, it isn't just your imagination.)

I could go on for days discussing the data showing the benefits of hormone replacement therapy, but you can find that information elsewhere. My goal here is to discuss clinically based thyroid replacement. But since estrogen is so vital to a woman's body and its deficiency causes so much dysfunction, it needed to be addressed to some degree here. I would again refer you to Dr. Bluming's excellent book *Estrogen Matters.*[19] It's one of the best and most comprehensive recent discussions that I have seen on the topic of HRT.

Remember, as an oncologist, Dr. Bluming has treated breast cancer patients for decades, so he should know what he is talking about. And he states clearly that the presence of breast cancer should not be considered a contraindication to using HRT.

I wish all medical students were assigned to read Dr. Bluming's book. It would teach them that replacing estrogen is usually very beneficial and rarely harmful, contrary to the current popular dogma. Of course, it would be a struggle of mammoth proportions to find time to assign books on clinical medicine in between all the questionably important topics currently taught in medical schools.

Take a look at the NYU Long Island School of Medicine's 3-year "Learning Community" curriculum,[20] which focuses on teaching moral reasoning and ethical analysis, "exploring medical humanities and social sciences," and training their students how to "form a professional identity." Unfortunately, they're not the only med school whose curriculum leaves out a solid understanding of hormonal physiology, which makes books like *Estrogen Matters* and my book even more important!

CHAPTER 4: FATIGUE, LOW ENERGY, AND SLEEP PROBLEMS

"Tired, but not the kind of tired that sleep fixes."
~ Maureen Johnson

In survey after survey, when asked about the worst symptoms of hypothyroidism, women consistently rate fatigue as number one. Underlying the fatigue in many hypothyroid patients are sleep disorders and problems that make it difficult or impossible to get restorative sleep. Fatigue and sleep-related issues are prevalent in hypothyroidism – but also very treatable!

FATIGUE AND LOW ENERGY

During my work with hypothyroid patients, at least 95% identified fatigue as one of their primary symptoms. Those who didn't list fatigue as a symptom were often over-compensators – women who are amazingly skilled at living with and pushing through their symptoms. In some cases, they were compulsive exercisers.

A perfect example of this was an athletic German woman I saw years ago, who was both a breast cancer survivor and a competitive runner. She had a remarkable "can-do" attitude and was able to push through her fatigue to compete in races quite successfully, despite having untreated hypothyroidism. Nonetheless, when we realized that she had symptoms of hypothyroidism and treated her,

her race times improved, and she started winning even more races! We were both quite pleased with that outcome!

Some women have also adapted and, for example, are so used to being extraordinarily tired that they consider it completely normal to need an afternoon nap just to make it through dinner. Some decline slowly, find themselves napping more frequently, and avoid various activities because they are too tired. Eventually, some women start withdrawing and avoiding most social interactions, becoming more depressed. Since all these symptoms are so intertwined, separating them from each other is difficult. The good news is that the same treatment will address all these symptoms concurrently.

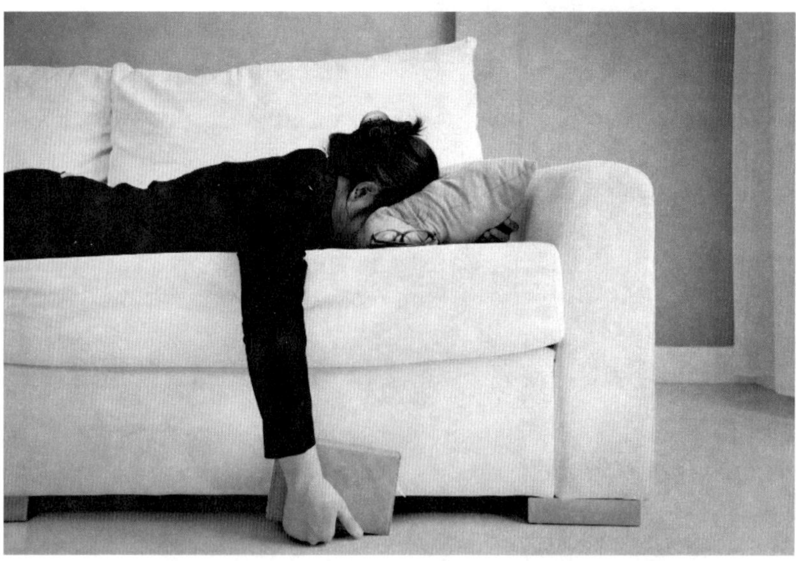

Most patients with fatigue due to hypothyroidism aren't compulsive athletes; they are just plain tired. Since standard medical care has no cure to offer them, they do whatever they can to get through their day. That may include frequent naps, early bedtimes, avoiding evening activities, use of caffeine, energy drinks, nicotine, Adderall, or other stimulant drugs. Occasionally they even have to quit work because they are too tired to get through a workday. Once this fatigue is adequately treated with thyroid, they often say they feel like they have their life back, which is immensely gratifying.

CHRONIC FATIGUE SYNDROME

Chronic Fatigue Syndrome started with the name "Chronic Epstein Barr Virus" in the mid-1980s. After an outbreak in Lake Tahoe in the late 1980s where no Epstein Barr virus was detected, the condition earned the new name Chronic Fatigue Syndrome, or CFS.

CFS is characterized by extreme fatigue, muscle pain, achy joints, headaches, poor concentration, memory issues, poor sleep quality, exercise intolerance, depression, and a sore throat.

In the 1950s, when a woman with significant fatigue went to her doctor, she was likely to be correctly diagnosed as hypothyroid based on her signs and symptoms. Then, her symptoms usually resolved with thyroid hormone replacement, and she was essentially cured. Since the 1980s, if the same woman went to her doctor with the same symptoms, the diagnosis and outcome will be very different. This time a TSH will be ordered which will most likely be "normal," which then "rules out" the possible diagnosis of hypothyroidism. Therefore, she was more likely to be diagnosed with depression, prescribed an antidepressant or mood stabilizer, or diagnosed with CFS or fibromyalgia, which have no definitive treatments, and still don't to this day. Since no good cure is offered, she may later end up unable to work, in a wheelchair, tied to a CPAP machine, on disability, hopeless and possibly suicidal, and taking a laundry list of various expensive medications that only partially treat her many and gradually worsening symptoms.

It's no coincidence that the symptoms of CFS are almost identical to hypothyroidism. It's also no coincidence that the prevalence of CFS has grown at the same time as the reliance on TSH for diagnosing and treating hypothyroidism has taken hold of the medical profession.

I'm not suggesting that every case of CFS will respond to thyroid hormone treatment. But, given how debilitating the condition can be, and the limited options available that have even a remote chance of resolving symptoms, I feel like it's fair to say that most CFS patients deserve a safely administered trial of thyroid hormone to see if it will help resolve their CFS symptoms.

SLEEP PROBLEMS AND DISORDERS

Hypothyroid patients *rarely* sleep well, making sleep another considerable challenge. Lab tests such as free T3, free T4, and TSH don't detect sleep problems. But when asked, most women with hypothyroidism will admit that they are experiencing persistent and disabling sleep problems. Consequently, they wake up tired and become even more tired over the course of the day.

The problems fall into several categories. First, some women fall asleep quickly at bedtime but consistently wake up in the middle of the night. They are drowsy and can sleep at 3 p.m. but are wide awake at 3 a.m. This is because sleep is an active process and requires some energy expenditure. Since metabolism is suboptimal 24 hours a day in hypothyroidism, solid sleep (which requires some energy to maintain) is often unobtainable.

This problem is very common in women already on a once-a-day morning dose of thyroid hormone. The morning dose of thyroid hormone wears off in the middle of the afternoon, and no thyroid remains left at night to fuel sleep. (I often thought that if I had ever wanted to advertise my services on TV or radio, I would have run ads in the inexpensive 3 a.m. time slot. Talk about target marketing!) The solution, however, is simple: Dosing twice a day – morning at lunchtime – frequently resolves these sleep problems.

Second, some hypothyroid patients have difficulty falling asleep. These women are so tired after work that they fall asleep on the couch for a couple of hours at dinnertime, then wake up at 9 p.m. for their evening. Often, these women have significant anxiety, so they report that their mind keeps racing when they go to bed and thus can't fall asleep. This issue also seems to be a bit more common in teenagers, who have shifted circadian rhythms, and ever-present cell phones to distract them at bedtime. The solution here is twofold. First, adding a lunchtime dose will often fix the afternoon slump, help prevent afternoon naps, and even somewhat reduce nighttime anxiety and mind racing. Second, it's important to avoid cell phones at bedtime. (But how to best extract a cell phone from the hands of a teenager is a task way above my pay grade!)

Finally, some women have more significant sleep disorders. Standard medicine currently treats a "sleep disorder" or "sleep apnea" as a disease, not a symptom of underlying hypothyroidism. Interestingly, many patients who came to me for their hypothyroidism had such bad issues with sleep that they have already had sleep studies done. In a sleep study, the patient tries to sleep, usually at a sleep lab, and a "sleep expert" watches them sleep and measures various things like blood oxygen level and whether or not the patient is achieving REM sleep. According to "The Sleep Blog" at www.sleepdr.com,[21] the average cost of one sleep study ranges from $300 to $3000. But some patients report the costs of these studies can be as high as $7,000 to $8,000! A variety of sleep problems can be detected during a sleep study, but the most common one is sleep apnea, and the usual treatments prescribed are sleeping pills and CPAP machines.

In sleep apnea, breathing is slowed or obstructed and sometimes stops during sleep, sometimes for several seconds or more, multiple times per night. This situation can be quite damaging to the tissues since interrupted breathing causes an interruption in the supply of oxygen getting to the tissues. Cells can't function optimally or even survive without oxygen. Apnea is associated with an increased risk of obesity, heart disease, increased mortality, and decreased brain function. Apnea is also, no surprise, *a symptom of untreated or poorly treated hypothyroidism!*

We know that there's a direct link between hypothyroidism and apnea. In 1983, Millman, Bevilacqua, Peterson, and Pack[22] reported on the case of a 45-year-old male patient who developed sleep apnea after being diagnosed with hypothyroidism. According to their account:

> *"In response to levothyroxine therapy, the patient became euthyroid, and the apneic phenomenon disappeared. Previous reports have suggested that hypothyroidism can produce obstructive sleep apnea from either narrowing of the upper airway…. or from abnormalities in ventilatory control."*

A few years later, in 1988, Kittle and Chaudhary wrote:[23] "Thyroid deficiency states are now a well-recognized cause of the sleep apnea syndrome." They go on to state that "The definitive therapy is thyroid hormone replacement, which has been shown to diminish or completely eliminate apneic episodes and arterial oxygen desaturation, as well as to effect many improvements in sleep patterns and overall sleep efficiency." They conclude, "Thyroid replacement therapy seems logical for the treatment of sleep apnea in patients with previously unrecognized subclinical hypothyroidism."

Hira and Sibal also discussed this association between hypothyroidism and sleep apnea in their 1999 publication, "An association of sleep apnea among patients with untreated hypothyroidism."[24] These researchers studied 20 consecutive hypothyroid patients with obstructive sleep apnea syndrome before and after initiating thyroid replacement. They found that sleep quality improved either wholly or partially in 19 of the 20 patients. They concluded that "there is a high incidence of sleep apnea among hypothyroid patients. Thyroxine treatment could achieve disappearance of these apneas in a majority of them."

Despite the widespread evidence that sleep apnea responds well to thyroid replacement, an article published in 1988 by RR Grunstein and an Australian researcher named Dr. Colin Edward Sullivan[25] attempted to deny this association. Their findings completely denied the benefits of using thyroid hormone to treat sleep issues. They even warned about the potential risks of using thyroid to improve sleep quality:

> *"Our experience suggests that the apnea index does not decrease significantly in all patients with hypothyroidism and sleep apnea when euthyroidism is achieved.... Treatment of hypothyroidism in the presence of sleep apnea is potentially hazardous and may lead to cardiovascular complications. Management by a combination of CPAP [a device that creates Continuous Positive Airway Pressure] and low-dose thyroxine is helpful in this situation."*

What do you think the authors meant by saying "when euthyroidism is achieved?" My wild guess is that it was defined by a specific TSH value or range and not by achieving complete resolution of hypothyroid symptoms. Nonetheless, it seemed strange that their results differed from the results of the other researchers.

To determine the reason for this discrepancy, I did a quick internet search and found that Dr. Sullivan *invented* nasal CPAP technology in 1980. He and his company, ResMed, have made hundreds of millions of dollars from his patented technology. Is it any wonder why he might downplay the benefits of thyroid for treating sleep disorders when the alternative is to prescribe technology that makes his company hundreds of millions of dollars? Welcome to the world of modern medical research!

Despite all the links between hypothyroidism and sleep apnea, the standard treatments for apnea have nothing to do with the thyroid. There are devices, including CPAP (continuous positive airway pressure), bi-level positive airway pressure (BPAP, or BiPap), various oral appliances designed to keep the airway open, and a computerized ventilator called "adaptive servo-ventilation" or ASV. Apnea sufferers may be advised to lose weight, avoid alcohol and smoking, sleep on their sides instead of the back, and get a special adjustable bed or pillow. In some cases, surgical procedures – and most of them are *extremely* painful – are recommended to open the upper airway. The most common surgery is uvulopalatopharyngoplasty (UPPP), and it's like removing the core of an apple if the back of your throat is the apple. Ouch!

Meanwhile, it's clear that replacing thyroid is the easiest, most physiologic, and it's likely the most effective treatment for sleep apnea.

As mentioned above, sleep apnea can be due to partial obstruction of the upper airway, called "obstructive sleep apnea," or decreased central stimulation of our breathing process. And as one would expect, treatments address both of these mechanisms – usually separately. Thyroid hormone replacement addresses *both* causes by reducing any tissue swelling that may be present in the oral pharynx (as it does in the rest of the body) *and* by stimulating the nervous system directly to drive the respiratory musculature.

But getting the dose high enough, but not too high, is critical, and giving a second dose at lunchtime is almost always required to attain solid, uninterrupted sleep at night. If the lunch dose is too high, the patient will find it harder to fall asleep, may wake up early in the morning for the day, and find it hard to fall back asleep. As with other symptoms of the central nervous system, I usually start with twice a day T4 to address poor sleep.

Everyone with sleep apnea won't have a complete cure with robust thyroid hormone replacement, but the fact is that many do. But before pushing these patients towards cumbersome CPAP and BPAP devices or costly, invasive, and painful apnea surgery, shouldn't they receive a trial of thyroid hormone? I think they should!

Also, don't forget that some sleep problems result from hot flashes or night sweats. See Chapter 3 for information about addressing estrogen levels concurrently with optimal thyroid treatment.

CHAPTER 5: BONE AND MUSCLE HEALTH

"We sometimes forget that bone is more than just a collection of calcium crystals. Bone is active, living tissue, continually remodeling itself and constantly participating in a wide range of biochemical reactions."
~ Alan Gaby, MD
From his book 'Preventing and Reversing Osteoporosis'[26]

Hypothyroidism generally does not adversely affect bone density unless it is so severe that it disrupts gastrointestinal (GI) function to the point of causing malnutrition. Many hypothyroid women have unusually dense bones, likely due to poor clearance of estrogen, testosterone, and DHEA (dehydroepiandrosterone, made in the adrenal glands) from the bloodstream, which all tend to stimulate the growth of bone. But thyroid replacement can cause bone loss if that replacement is excessive and prolonged. In addition, estrogen deficiency due to menopause is a major contributor to bone loss. Consequently, when dealing with these hormonal deficiencies, it's wise to understand how these hormones affect our bones.

In contrast, muscle health and strength directly depend on good thyroid function. Many women with hypothyroidism struggle with muscle weakness and other health complications. Let's take a look at some of these essential connections.

BONE EFFECTS AND OSTEOPOROSIS

One of the adverse effects of *hyper*thyroidism, whether spontaneous or iatrogenic (due to overmedication), is the risk of osteoporosis. I once had a patient whose prior hyperthyroidism had been so poorly controlled by her doctors that her spine was curved forward at almost a 90-degree angle due to significant lumbar osteoporosis and collapse of multiple vertebral bodies. In order to see ahead when walking, she had to severely hyperextend her neck backward and upward so that her eyes were facing forward and not facing the ground! Another elderly menopausal patient of petite stature who had always shunned HRT had such bad osteoporosis that she had to wear a corset around her torso, like an exoskeleton, to keep herself upright. I don't remember if she had a history of hyperthyroidism, but the image of her wearing her exoskeleton corset will never escape my memory.

Sadly, the problem with osteoporosis is that once the bone is gone, it's gone, and you really can't do much to bring it back entirely. Some drugs like bisphosphonates, Prolia, and Forteo will increase bone density a bit, but they generally can only be used safely for a few years and have some significant risks. Consequently, I have always taken extra care to never contribute to bone loss by giving too much thyroid and doing whatever I can to help women preserve bone. That's why I had all my patients do periodic bone density assessments while on thyroid hormone, particularly if the TSH level is low or suppressed.

Many years ago, when I started treating patients with thyroid hormone, I still believed that a suppressed TSH meant that the patient was overdosed and would lose bone. So, like the endocrinologists taught me, if a patient's TSH became suppressed on the dose that made their symptoms go away – and most did – I would reduce the patient's dose of thyroid to normalize the TSH. I believed bone loss would occur if the TSH level were below the "normal range." The only patient with a suppressed TSH that I didn't do this to was myself. Even though my TSH was close to 0.0, I figured I knew how my body was responding to my dose, I had no symptoms of overdose, and I was not going to sue myself if I lost bone. I would simply do follow-up bone density studies to see if I had any bone loss.

Lo and behold, despite my 0.0 TSH, my follow-up bone density showed no bone loss at all! Imagine that! The dose that was relieving all my symptoms of hypothyroidism – and not causing any clinical symptoms or signs of overdose – was *also* not causing bone loss! That's when I realized that the TSH test was truly worthless. A normal TSH does not mean you aren't hypothyroid, and a completely suppressed TSH does not mean you are overdosed. The only good it does is for the drug industry: It keeps doctors from treating hypothyroid patients adequately, so they continue to prescribe a bunch of other drugs to treat all the symptoms that are left unresolved. It's quite diabolical, actually.

After realizing that I wasn't losing bone with my suppressed TSH, I began to allow my patients to stay on the doses that had resolved all their symptoms, usually with a TSH level near 0. I asked all of them to have regular bone density tests to prove that we were not causing bone loss. Not surprisingly, their results were the same as my results. Most of my patients who were well replaced and had no symptoms or signs of overdose – even with a TSH of 0.0 – were not losing bone. Great news! I continued to have my patients with a suppressed TSH level – again, most of them fit into this category – get regular bone density tests since I never want to take the chance that I could be causing them to lose bone mass. Osteoporosis is preventable, and we should always do whatever we can to prevent it.

Of course, some women did have some bone loss, and when that occurred, I would investigate possible causes of that loss which include the following:

- Too much thyroid replacement
- Too little estrogen (failure to replace estrogen after menopause or use of estrogen blockers)
- Inadequate Vitamin D
- Being underweight for years
- Chronic steroid use

- Smoking
- Malnutrition (due to malabsorption from gluten intolerance, chronic diarrhea, gastric bypass surgery, anorexia, antacids)
- Hyperparathyroidism
- Hypoadrenalism

Once the most likely factors causing or allowing bone loss have been identified, treatment must be adjusted to address those problems. But the dose must be lowered if a woman is even slightly overdosed with thyroid. If a woman has subtle symptoms of estrogen deficiency – like occasional mild night sweats, the absence of any breast sensitivity, or a low serum estradiol level (I like it to be at least around 50 pg./ml or more) – the estrogen dose should be increased. If the total Vitamin D 25-OH level is under 40 to 50 ng/ml, I also recommend increasing that dose. If the serum calcium level is elevated and still elevated on the repeat test, I recommend a parathyroid hormone (PTH) test to evaluate for hyperparathyroidism.

If a woman is having gastrointestinal issues that are likely causing malabsorption, address those issues with a gluten-free diet, a multivitamin, or other appropriate interventions. If a woman is unusually thin, and she doesn't want to gain weight – and who does? – I recommend exercising while wearing a weight vest or a backpack full of books or water bottles to trick the bones into getting stronger. (Bones get denser if the weight they carry is increased.)

Osteoporosis drugs are rarely necessary when all possible causes of bone loss are properly assessed and addressed. And while it makes sense, sadly, this isn't the currently recommended standard of care for bone density issues. Instead, the standard routine is to order a DEXA bone density scan, find criteria that warrant a diagnosis of osteopenia or osteoporosis, and then reflexively prescribe one of the popular bone health drugs–usually the newest. I used that shotgun approach decades ago when Fosamax first came out, but as I got a little older and hopefully a bit wiser, I learned what I believe is a more thoughtful and better approach. I hope you think so too.

The most common causative factors I have found are usually lack of estrogen, lack of vitamin D, or other nutritional factors. Notice that the lack of a gym membership is not a significant risk factor. In my opinion, nutritional and hormonal factors are much more important than exercise. Once the cause of the bone loss is identified, we do whatever is needed to fix that factor. If a patient wishes to "do weights" at a gym, I always say, "be my guest," but let her know that exercise is not an adequate substitute for full estrogen replacement or healthy Vitamin D levels. I had a number of patients try to exercise regularly instead of taking HRT, which *never* worked. Without estrogen, they continued to lose bone.

I often told women that the most effective exercise to yield strong bones is to pick up an estrogen patch, pull the backing tabs off, and place the patch on their skin! The consequence of this approach was that very few of my patients had fractures or even needed any of the bone drugs that have become so popular, thanks to the recommendations of the National Osteoporosis Foundation. I even had one of my slender, very active, healthy 70-year-old long-term HRT patients fall through her attic floor to the floor below, and she didn't break a thing! She considered her fall as reassuring as a bone density test! I can't disagree with her.

We should also remember that hypothyroidism will often cause the bone density to be abnormally high in many cases. Thyroid hormone controls bone turnover, the process whereby osteoclasts chew up the surface of the bone, and the osteoblasts come in to lay down new bone where the old bone has been removed. It's very similar to the road maintenance teams that mill and resurface our roads. So, like our roads, bone is constantly being resurfaced to fix minor micro-fractures, like cracks in the road surface, so that they do not become major clinical fractures. This process keeps our bones strong. Bone turnover is also necessary during childhood, when bones grow and reshape themselves as we learn to walk upright. It's also necessary for the healing process if there is a fracture.

When thyroid is deficient, the resurfacing process slows down, particularly the osteoclast part, and the net result is that bone can accumulate. Also, if the patient is hypothyroid during her menstruating years, her estrogen level goes up, further feeding her bones. Finally, if one gains weight from having a sluggish metabolism, that creates an additional "weight bearing" effect on the skeleton whenever the patient is upright. It's not uncommon to see very high bone density results in patients who have been hypothyroid for many years. They will invariably claim that their high bone density is due to their years of going to the gym, but let's be honest: other factors are also very likely at play!

There's no reason to worry if a woman starts out with very high bone density and begins to go down a little bit with thyroid treatment. This is usually a sign that the original very high bone density was an abnormality, and the bone is returning to a more normal density. The changes should level out as the bone density approaches normal. When everything is done right – fully replacing estrogen, thyroid hormone, and Vitamin D – bone density will stabilize even as other women lose bone density after menopause. Of course, the goals are the absence of fractures and a bone density level above average, particularly as women age.

It's also fascinating that severe hypothyroidism can *cause* bone loss. I had a 12-year-old patient, Jenna, who weighed only 64 pounds and was never hungry due to gastroparesis (lack of gastrointestinal motility) caused by her severe hypothyroidism. Her bone density was very low before therapy because she was chronically malnourished. Girls and women who are severely hypothyroid usually eat very little because hypothyroidism slows their gastrointestinal function almost to a standstill. These ladies never feel like their stomach is empty, so they rarely feel hungry. If a woman only eats 500 to 700 calories a day – because that's all it takes to feel full – she is not consuming enough nutrients to build healthy and strong bones. So those girls and ladies who are extremely cold and tired, with a basal temperature around 96 or lower, will often be skinny and have fragile bones to match because they, and their bones, are literally starving.

When given the correct thyroid dose, they regain the function of their gastrointestinal tract and begin eating and absorbing the nutrients they need to build bone. In the case of Jenna, within 14 months after she started on thyroid hormone, her spine density increased by 21%, and she grew 4 inches in height.

Though it's widely known that hyperthyroidism can cause osteoporosis, it isn't widely known that hypothyroidism can cause low bone mass. However, I am happy to report that several relatively recent articles have finally discussed this effect. In 2014, Dominika Tuchendler and Marek Bolanowski[27] said that "both excess as well as deficiency of fT4 and fT3 can be potentially deleterious for bone tissue." Then in 2018, G R Williams and J H D Bassett[28] discussed the following:

> *"Thyroid hormones are essential for skeletal development and are important regulators of bone maintenance in adults. Childhood hypothyroidism causes delayed skeletal development, retarded linear growth and impaired bond mineral accrual.... Thyroid hormone replacement stimulates catch-up growth and bone maturation."*

This is exactly what I saw in sweet, young, cold, and tired Jenna with gastroparesis.

I encourage practitioners to look for this syndrome because it isn't uncommon in young women and also very elderly women with "the dwindles" that I discuss in Chapter 13. When physicians know how to recognize it, and are willing to fix it, a lot of good can be done for these ladies. Imagine how much pain, suffering, illness, and immobility can be prevented by fixing this malnutrition-inducing situation early in life! It's well worth the effort.

MUSCLE WEAKNESS, INCREASED VASCULAR RESISTANCE

Many hypothyroid patients complain of muscle weakness, lacking the muscle motor strength or endurance they previously enjoyed. In addition, I was taught in medical school that reflexes in a hypothyroid patient are slow to commence and resolve. Half a century ago, many researchers confirmed these phenomena in rats and human subjects. Below are a few of these studies.

In 1970, Gold, Spann, and Braunwald[29] reported the results of their research studying the function of the soleus muscles of rats that had had their thyroid glands ablated (myxedematous hypothyroid rats) compared to the function in normal (euthyroid) rats and to that of hyperthyroid rats. Upon stimulating the muscles of these three groups of rats, they found that the euthyroid and hyperthyroid rats had a similar response. Still, muscle response – both contracting and relaxing – was *much* slower in the hypothyroid rats. This study confirms what I heard from patients, time and time again.

In 1978, Flaim, Li, and Jefferson[30] studied rats who were hypothyroid after thyroidectomy. They found that the rate of muscle protein growth was reduced by 50% in the hypothyroid rats; replacing T4 reversed this reduction. This lack of muscle protein growth would explain why the 1970 finding that the muscles don't work as well during hypothyroidism, and how replacing thyroid treatment reverses this problem. How convenient!

Not surprisingly, a series of studies in the 1980s showed similar results in human subjects. In 1981, Wiles, Jones, and Edwards[31] published "The pathophysiology of muscle fatigue …in patients with thyroid dysfunction." Their research reported that:

> *"Muscle from hypothyroid patients, like cooled muscle, is slow in relaxing and showed a reduced energy requirement…fatigue is premature and associated with impaired excitation."*

(In plain English, muscles were slow to contract, slow to relax, and tired easily.)

In a related study in 1989, Zurcher et al.[32] studied both thigh muscle size and efficiency in hypothyroid, euthyroid, and hyperthyroid patients. They reported that:

> *"The muscle efficiency (total work output per cm2 muscle) increased in all patients after therapy [and] ... patients with thyroid dysfunction have altered muscle mass and diminished muscle efficiency."*

Finally, in 1984, Khaleeli and Edwards[33] reported the following:

> *"Measurements of quadriceps force revealed significant muscle weakness when comparison with 15 age matched healthy subjects was made (P less than 0.001). This weakness was often not evident on clinical examination...Weakness was slow to recover and seven patients remained weak at the end of the study despite being euthyroid for a mean period of 1 year, but strength increased modestly overall (P less than 0.01)."*

Unfortunately, the authors used the TSH to determine the dose of thyroid replacement in this study, which suggests to me that these patients were likely inadequately replaced. This would explain why their therapy's resolution of the weakness was incomplete. However, in my experience, the weakness entirely resolves when the thyroid is adequately replaced.

The effect of thyroid on smooth muscle is a bit different than its effect on striated (motor) muscle. In the case of motor muscle, thyroid hormone stimulates its growth and strength. In contrast, the impact of thyroid hormone on certain types of smooth muscle, i.e., the muscle fibers that surround our blood vessels and airways, is generally to cause relaxation. This effect was studied in 1989 by Ishikawa et al.,[34] who exposed strips of rabbit artery to T3 and T4. They found that both T3 and T4 caused the smooth muscle of the artery wall to relax. They concluded that "thyroid hormones act directly at the blood vessel wall to cause inhibition of the contractile process in vascular smooth muscle."

A few years later, in 1993, Ojamaa, Balkman, and Klein[35] studied vascular resistance in human subjects. They wrote that

> *"Systemic vascular resistance is uniformly decreased in both naturally occurring and experimental hyperthyroidism, and it's increased in thyroid hormone deficiency."*

Further, they noted that "vascular smooth muscle cell contraction is a major determinant of systemic vascular resistance." They specifically studied the effects of T3 and concluded the following:

> *"Our data indicate that triiodothyronine causes smooth muscle relaxation: this property may account for some of its marked effects on the cardiovascular system. As a novel vasodilatory agent, the potential therapeutic implications for triiodothyronine may be numerous."*

These researchers were essentially suggesting that T3 could be used to lower blood pressure. Little did these naïve researchers know that thyroid would be used only to normalize elevated TSH values and *not* for valuable functions such as lowering vascular resistance, thus normalizing elevated blood pressure. Why would we ever want to do that when we have so many man-made, expensive, and profitable anti-hypertensive drugs to choose from for that very same purpose? How foolish of them!

CHAPTER 6: CARDIOVASCULAR HEALTH

"Heart disease – not breast or any other cancer – is the number-one killer of women over age 65 and the second leading cause of death among women aged 45 to 64. Women account for 52 percent of the 80 million Americans who have heart disease and who die from heart disease and heart attacks."
~ Mache Seibel

The entire cardiovascular system relies on thyroid hormone to function well, and many conditions can result when women are hypothyroid. This chapter looks at high blood pressure, shortness of breath, pulse and heart rhythm irregularities, high cholesterol, and circulatory health.

HYPERTENSION

There's a clear association between hypothyroidism and hypertension, also known as high blood pressure. Quite a few research papers linking hypertension and hypothyroidism were written in the 1960s and 1970s. Sadly, only a few of those articles are available online. The oldest one I found was published in the UK in 1938 and is titled "Endocrinal Obesity (Hypothyroidism) with Oedema of the Legs, Osteoarthritis and Hypertension."[36] This was a case report of a 48-year-old woman who had difficulty walking due to pain and swelling of her legs and was, according to the article, "more or less confined to bed." She weighed 298 pounds and displayed multiple symptoms and signs of hypothyroidism. Her blood pressure was high at 190/115. No TSH level was available; the test hadn't been invented yet.

According to the research, the patient was treated with a "radiant heat bath; lymphatic massage; faradism to arms, legs, and abdomen. Later, remedial exercises and rowing machine." (Faradism is an outdated form of electrical current therapy that stimulates muscles.) She was also treated with diuretic suppositories, a salt-free 1,000 calorie low-carbohydrate diet, restricted fluids, and 120 mg (2 grains) of thyroid extract three times a day. (Note: That thyroid hormone dosage was about six times the standard dose that endocrinologists would use today.)

According to the article, the results were as follows:

> *"The patient has lost 5 stone [70 pounds] in weight, is able to walk well, and has an almost full range of movement of the upper and lower limbs which now show some signs of the shape of the ankles. The oedema has almost subsided. There is marked reduction in the measurements of ankles and calves."*

Unfortunately, this paper did not report the blood pressure after the patient had lost 70 pounds and could walk again, but I suspect it was much closer to normal. The other obvious problem with this report is that multiple interventions were used at once, so we can't definitively know which therapy yielded the benefit (though I suspect the thyroid was at the top of that list!)

A 1965 Canadian paper[37] described eight cases of myxedema, swelling, and fluid retention resulting from advanced hypothyroidism. Two of the patients studied presented with significant hypertension. According to the study, both patients "showed a marked fall in blood pressure with treatment of the myxedema." The first of the two was a 44-year-old woman with symptoms including severe headaches, visual changes, and blood pressure ranging from 200-240/160-180. After treatment with 200 mg (3.3 grains) of natural desiccated thyroid per day, her headaches resolved, her vision improved, and her blood pressure dropped to 150/100. The second woman was a 54-year-old housewife with six years of shortness of breath, facial puffiness, and other symptoms, including blood pressure of 200/115. The dose that made her feel better was ultimately 300 mg (5 grains) of NDT daily. This dose dropped her blood pressure to 140/80.

The authors noted that "hypertension is common in patients with myxedema." They referenced a 1933 paper by Lerman, Clark, and Means[38] that reported on 14 patients with myxedema and hypertension. After treatment of those patients with thyroid, "five developed normal blood pressure and six had a fall in blood pressure, but not to normal levels." They wisely concluded that when myxedema and hypertension are present simultaneously, the best approach is to treat the thyroid deficiency first because the blood pressure may very well normalize, making blood pressure treatment unnecessary.

I also found that hypertension in many of my patients resolved with thyroid treatment. But remember that these therapeutic doses used in the 1930s – and the doses I used with my patients – are larger than the tiny doses used today to treat abnormal TSH tests. This explains why modern doctors who grew up as TSH believers aren't aware of the therapeutic benefit of thyroid hormone for hypertension. Unfortunately, the doses they commonly prescribe these days are simply too small to yield significant benefits for patients with hypertension.

In the early 1980s, several papers were published linking hypothyroidism with hypertension. Okamura, Inoue, Shiroozu, et al. published a study in 1980[39] that evaluated the long-term health of patients who had had Graves' disease more than 10 years earlier, and who were clinically hypothyroid at the time of the study. The researchers reported that the "incidence of hypertension seemed to be significantly higher in the TSH-elevated euthyroid group compared with the TSH-nonelevated patients." In this case, patients were described as "euthyroid" because their TSH levels fell within the normal range.

Later that year, Bing, Briggs, and Burden et al. published a paper[40] out of Oxford, documenting "six patients with hypothyroidism and hypertension whose blood pressure fell to normal when treated with thyroxine." As in the Lerman study of 1933, these authors concluded that "hypertension in the hypothyroid patients only requires further evaluation if it persists after adequate treatment with thyroxine."

Finally, in 1983, when I finished my residency, Saito, Ito, and Saruta published a study in the journal *Hypertension*[41] "to study whether there is an association between hypertension and hypothyroidism… in 477 female patients with chronic thyroiditis." About two-thirds of the subjects had normal TSH tests, and one-third had elevated TSH values. Once again, these researchers found that blood pressure, particularly diastolic blood pressure, was higher in hypothyroid patients than in those with normal thyroid levels. Also, as in the other studies, adequate treatment resolved hypertension. According to the researchers:

> *"Adequate thyroid hormone replacement therapy for an average 14.8 months in 14 patients resulted in a normalization of thyroid function and a reduction of blood pressure (p less than 0.01). In four who showed no change in thyroid function due to inadequate replacement therapy, blood pressure remained elevated. These results suggest a close association between hypertension and hypothyroidism."*

These studies, which took place over half a century, consistently showed a positive association between hypothyroidism and hypertension and that optimal thyroid replacement could normalize elevated blood pressure. Still, most doctors today are unaware of any association between the two. Sure, they're often aware that hyperthyroidism and thyroid hormone *overdose* can cause hypertension, but few know that a lack of thyroid hormone can do the same. Sometimes I just have to shake my head at the quality of medical training these days.

SHORTNESS OF BREATH

Breathing requires the smooth muscles that encircle the airways to relax, along with fully functional diaphragm and chest wall muscles to expand and contract the lungs. When those muscles don't work correctly, air doesn't move easily, and breathing is impaired, resulting in shortness of breath. As we discussed in Chapter 5, muscle function is impaired in hypothyroidism. Thus, it's no surprise that hypothyroid women often complain of shortness of breath and exercise intolerance.

A literature review reveals many articles discussing the relationship between hypothyroidism and shortness of breath. A group of Japanese researchers added to our understanding of this symptom in a 1983 paper by Yamamoto et al.[42] that revealed that "arterial blood analysis indicated a frequent incidence of hypoxia in hypothyroidism. The incidence of hypoxia was 69%. The hypoxia was improved by thyroxine replacement therapy." (Hypoxia is a low blood oxygen level, also known as oxygen deficiency.)

The presence of hypoxia in hypothyroid patients is likely due to dysfunction of the muscles that generate proper air movement in the lungs. The research shows that thyroid deficiency leads to respiratory muscle dysfunction, which, in turn, impedes air flow and gas exchange in the lungs. Consequently, this study showed that the percentage of oxygen in the blood is reduced. The consequence of that reduction in oxygen concentration is the shortness of breath experienced by some hypothyroid patients.

When breathing is impaired by hypothyroid muscle dysfunction, not only is oxygen (O_2) reduced but carbon dioxide (CO_2) is increased in the bloodstream. A study by Ladenson, Goldenheim, and Ridgway in 1988[43] evaluated the ventilatory responses to the presence of reduced O_2 and increased CO_2 among 38 hypothyroid patients. They found hypothyroid patients "were significantly more likely to have impaired ventilatory responses." And, as we would predict, therapy with thyroid replacement reversed these impairments. They reported:

> *"In seven of nine patients with abnormal pretreatment hypercapnic [too much CO_2 in the blood] responses, normal ventilatory responsiveness was restored after one week of therapy……thyroid hormone therapy for one week reverses impaired ventilatory responses in hypothyroidism."*

In 1985, Italian researchers[44] found the same results. They concluded, "hypercapnic ventilatory drive is blunted by short-term hypothyroidism and normalizes following replacement therapy."

Muscle dysfunction isn't the only thing contributing to respiratory dysfunction and shortness of breath in hypothyroid patients. Delay in nerve conduction time is also a contributor. In 1988 Laroche, Cairns et al.[45] studied a 58-year-old woman with recurrent chest infections, breathlessness, and orthopnea. (Orthopnea is breathlessness when lying down that is relieved when sitting or standing.) She also complained of tiredness and aching limbs. Her TSH was above 50, suggesting profound hypothyroidism. Pulmonary function tests revealed "severe bilateral diaphragm weakness…demonstrated by a greatly reduced maximal transdiaphragmatic pressure." In addition, nerve conduction studies demonstrated that impulses going down the phrenic nerves – the nerves that take messages from the brain to the diaphragm – were prolonged on both sides. Happily – and no surprise – thyroid replacement reversed both issues.

> *"Three months after starting treatment with thyroxine she had become euthyroid, and phrenic nerve conduction times and PDI relaxation rates had returned to normal. Maximal respiratory pressures, vital capacity, and maximal voluntary ventilation improved progressively on treatment…. We conclude that hypothyroidism may present with breathlessness due to respiratory muscle weakness and/or phrenic nerve neuropathy and is reversible with treatment."*

Not only is there a direct correlation between pulmonary dysfunction and hypothyroidism, but there is also a positive correlation between the degree of pulmonary dysfunction and the degree of TSH elevation. A 1992 study by Siafakas, Salesiotou, and Filaditaki et al.[46] investigated respiratory muscle strength in patients with hypothyroidism and compared their findings to the degree of TSH elevation. Among other things, they measured peak inspiration (PImax) and peak expiration (PEmax). The results were not surprising:

> *"a highly significant linear relationship was found between PImax and TSH and between PEmax and TSH…. We conclude that hypothyroidism affects respiratory muscle strength and that this weakness is linearly related to thyroid hormone levels. Respiratory muscle weakness is present in both inspiratory and expiratory muscles and is reversible with treatment."*

Finally, in 2017, a well-done Egyptian study by Sadek, Khalifa, and Azoz[47] confirmed the findings of the prior researchers that showed an association between hypothyroidism and diminished lung function. These authors did a case-controlled study of 42 subjects with newly diagnosed hypothyroidism, comparing them to 12 age and weight-matched control subjects. All subjects had TSH levels above 6 and low free T4 values. All subjects and the controls had multiple pulmonary function measurements performed at rest and with exercise. Their conclusions were as follows:

> *"Hypothyroidism has a significant effect both in resting PFTs [pulmonary function tests] and exercise testing parameters even in its early stage, so we recommend early intervention in cases of hypothyroidism with strict observation of pulmonary function and exercise tolerance.*
>
> *The strength of the study is that our patients were newly diagnosed with overt hypothyroidism with nil thyroid replacement therapy, our patients had no other comorbidities, and hence pulmonary exercise effects were solely related to low thyroid hormone levels."*

These authors demonstrated a relationship between hypothyroidism and lung dysfunction that causes shortness of breath at rest and exercise intolerance. This particular article also includes a helpful review of some of the literature which you might find of interest if you want to learn more specifics about the thyroid's effect on pulmonary function

The bottom line is that our ability to breathe and oxygenate our blood, like all other body functions, is directly dependent on optimal thyroid function. Sub-par thyroid function often results in the sensation of shortness of breath and exercise intolerance. So, we have yet one more important argument in favor of full thyroid hormone replacement. Giving only enough thyroid to normalize the TSH is simply not good enough and can leave patients still feeling short of breath.

SLOW PULSE AND ARRHYTHMIAS

It's also important to look at the impact of thyroid hormone directly on the heart. As with other organs, thyroid hormone drives the heart's function just as it drives the function of everything else in a mammal's body. If your body were an automobile, thyroid hormone would be the accelerator pedal. Just as your car does not run well if there is too little pressure on the accelerator pedal, inadequate thyroid function significantly affects the cardiovascular system. The first and most obvious effect is on the pulse. Hyperthyroidism is associated with an elevated pulse, and hypothyroidism often causes a low pulse.

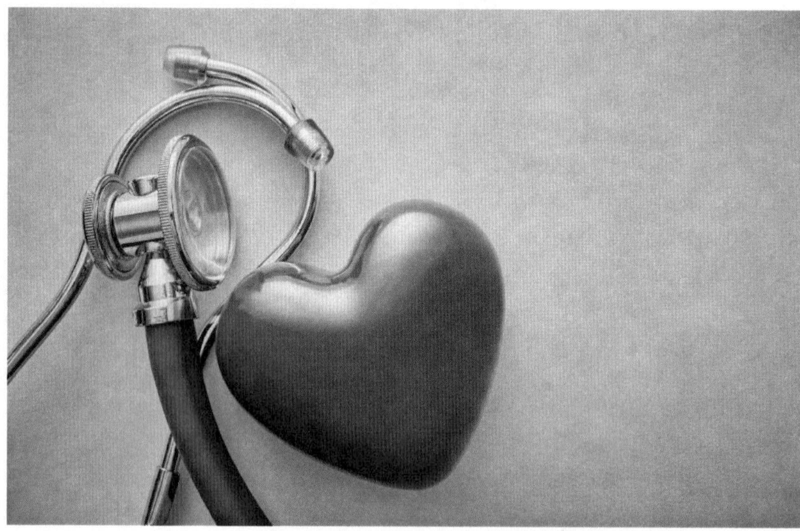

As with blood pressure, it again seems that most doctors are aware of the former association, but few are aware of the latter. I once had a 200-pound patient who did no regular exercise tell me that another physician had told her that he thought she was in excellent cardiovascular shape because her pulse was often in the 50s. Yikes! Indeed, all that physician had learned during their training was that low pulse rate is present in people with very efficient cardiovascular function. No one had taught him that a low pulse is also a classic sign of low metabolic rate, i.e., low thyroid function. Exceptionally good cardiovascular conditioning is one cause of a low pulse but certainly not the most common cause. This is another example of how plain old common sense and reason seem to have gone the way of the dinosaurs when it comes to clinical diagnosis.

Not everyone with hypothyroidism has a low pulse, but it's a valuable clue if they do. The pulse will likely climb back into a normal range when the correct replacement dose is found. I generally like to see an average resting evening pulse somewhere between 65 and 85 in most women once they're on the correct dose of thyroid. Of course, there are exceptions, particularly if someone is also a marathon runner or hypoadrenal, but generally, that seems to be a good range for a pulse. I usually expect T4 to raise the pulse more than T3, but both can do so.

Conversely, it's *very important* to ensure the pulse does not go too high while on thyroid hormone replacement. Why? An elevated pulse can be a sign that the dose is too high! Overstimulating the heart can do significant harm, just like racing the engine in your car can eventually burn up your engine. I always encouraged my patients to monitor their resting evening pulse every day, preferably using their fingers instead of an electronic device, so they can detect irregularities in the rhythm as well as the rate as soon as they might first appear.

I asked them to do this in the evening when the effects of the day's doses would likely be peaking. Daily pulse monitoring helped ensure that my patients did not end up in an emergency room with atrial fibrillation. I warned them that I would be asking what their pulse had been whenever we talked. I sometimes even threatened them with "pulse-shaming" if they weren't taking their pulse and stressed the importance of self-monitoring the pulse. It's an essential and simple safety measure, and there is really no valid excuse for not self-monitoring the pulse rate.

As for Fitbits and other electronic pulse monitoring devices, I have found that some of them do not pick up irregular rhythms. If the rhythm is irregular, the device may read out a perfectly normal pulse. This happened to me with one patient whose Fitbit wristband showed a pulse of 72, but when I felt her pulse manually, it was highly irregular. For that reason, I asked patients with such devices to also regularly feel their pulse with their fingers to ensure the rhythm is regular. If they really prefer to depend solely on technology, the Kardia Mobile is a $99 device that works with their cell phone to do a mini-EKG whenever they want. The Kardia Mobile is a handy little tool for women who occasionally experience an irregular heart rate.

In summary, as briefly discussed earlier, thyroid directly affects the heart rate, and great care should be taken to ensure that the pulse stays in range and the rhythm stays regular. Too low or too high a pulse are both a problem. That's why daily monitoring is essential because one of the most significant adverse events that can occur with thyroid overdose is atrial fibrillation or other arrhythmias. If allowed to persist long enough, these rhythm irregularities can cause intra-cardiac clot formation, where blood clots can form in the heart chambers. These clots can, in turn, send emboli downstream, which can cause strokes, heart attacks, and even death. Do not ignore this!!!

HIGH CHOLESTEROL, ATHEROSCLEROSIS, AND METABOLIC SYNDROME

There's another way that thyroid hormone affects the cardiovascular system. It's not well known today, but there's an inverse association between thyroid function and cholesterol. The higher the thyroid function, the lower the cholesterol level. This was common knowledge decades ago, but this important association is no longer taught in medical school. Back in the 1970s, in medical school, I certainly wasn't taught that hypothyroidism causes high cholesterol and that you can lower cholesterol by replacing thyroid hormone. Yet, this association was well documented in the medical literature back in the 1960s and before. Indeed, the medical literature from the 1940s through the 1960s is filled with studies linking thyroid function and serum cholesterol levels.

For example, an article published in 1959 by Yale researchers John Peters and Evelyn Man[48] explains that:

> *"The discovery that serum cholesterol was elevated in myxedema and experimental hypothyroidism led to the clinical use of cholesterol measurements as a diagnostic aid…there proved to be a statistical inverse correlation between serum cholesterol and thyroid activity."*

We'll discuss this in more detail in Chapter 10 when we discuss thyroid's effect on the liver.

In addition, some research published during that time discussed the ability of thyroid hormone to inhibit the accumulation of plaque, as one might predict would happen when using a substance that has been shown to lower cholesterol. As far back as 1933, we can find a study by KB Turner[49] at Columbia University which showed that:

> *"Whole thyroid gland when administered simultaneously with cholesterol prevented the atheromatous changes produced by the latter in the aorta of rabbits."*

Fascinating! Well, what about humans? Does it also inhibit plaque in humans? Good question. The answer is yes; it apparently does.

Dr. Broda Barnes discussed this association thoroughly in his 1976 book, *Solved: The Riddle of Heart Attacks.*[50] Dr. Barnes discussed autopsy data from Austria showing much more atherosclerosis in the corpses of people who died from tuberculosis (TB) compared to those who did not have TB. This was a time when TB was the most common cause of death in this country. Dr. Barnes argued that hypothyroidism made people more prone to infections like TB because thyroid deficiency impaired the immune system. It also resulted in plaque. Once treatments for TB were identified and people who were prone to TB were no longer dying of their infections, they later died of heart disease. When we learned how to control TB, heart disease became the number one cause of death in the US.

Many of these findings concerning thyroid hormone replacement's ability to prevent heart disease by inhibiting plaque formation are also discussed in Dr. Barnes's other book, *Hypothyroidism, the Unsuspected Illness.*[51] I recently contacted a very prominent and highly regarded research cardiologist[52] about the possibility of using thyroid hormone to prevent or even reverse atherosclerosis. He rejected the idea based on a study done in the late '60s called the Coronary Drug Project.[53]

In that study, dextrothyroxine (D-thyroxine) at a dose of 6 mg per day (6,000 mcg) was given to male subjects and caused "untoward pro-arrhythmias leading to early termination" of the study. (D-thyroxine was a thyroid replacement and cholesterol-lowering drug pulled from the market due to cardiac-related side effects. I'm not sure how D-thyroxine compares to levothyroxine in clinical efficacy at the cellular level but giving the same large dose to a group of randomly selected men – who may or may not have had signs and symptoms of hypothyroidism – isn't exactly what I would call a fair trial. That would be like doing a study giving 200 units of insulin to a bunch of random subjects who may or may not be diabetic and concluding that insulin therapy does not reduce the morbidity of diabetes. (Fortunately, they did not study insulin in the Coronary Drug Project. Using that shotgun approach, they would have ended up killing a lot of people.) Happily, thyroid is a lot more forgiving than insulin for those subjects!

It's almost as if the researchers who designed this study were purposely using the wrong dose of the wrong drug in the wrong subjects to prove that thyroid replacement did not help prevent plaque. No, surely that could never happen!! All medical research is simply designed to find the truth, right? Perhaps not, particularly when studying an inexpensive medicine that can prevent a very profitable and common disease.

Nonetheless, it's quite disappointing that this highly respected research cardiologist would entirely discount the potential benefits of properly done thyroid replacement in patients with signs and symptoms of hypothyroidism as a way to lower cholesterol and inhibit plaque accumulation. He's a smart guy, so perhaps I'll try discussing it with him again in the future!

Most interest in studying thyroid replacement as a prevention for heart disease comes from outside the US. For example, in 1994, a group out of Saitama Medical University in Japan published a study entitled "Disturbed lipid metabolism in patients with subclinical hypothyroidism: effect of L-thyroxine therapy."[54] Authors Miura, Iitaka, and Yoshimura et al. found that two months of "L-4 [levothyroxine] therapy significantly decreased the serum level of … total cholesterol (TC; P<.02)." The list of articles that have cited this important Japanese study reads like the roll call at the United Nations, yet US research centers have rarely cited this work. That's unfortunate and quite telling.

In 2015, another very interesting paper from Belgrade, Serbia, entitled "Effects of Levothyroxine Replacement Therapy on Parameters of Metabolic Syndrome and Atherosclerosis in Hypothyroid Patients: A Prospective Pilot Study."[55] Here Zoran Gluvic, Emina Sudar, and Jelena Tica et al. sought to study the effects of levothyroxine replacement therapy on various parameters of atherosclerosis and what is now called "metabolic syndrome" in 30 female patients. They found that 3 months of levothyroxine replacement caused a significant reduction in body mass index, blood pressure, total cholesterol, LDL-C, and IMCT (intima-media complex thickness).

Isn't that fascinating?! This study demonstrated that most abnormalities found in "metabolic syndrome" can be reversed with thyroid replacement. Quelle surprise, as the French would say!

The term "metabolic syndrome" was used and popularized back in 1977 by Herman Haller[56] when he was studying the risk factors for atherosclerotic cardiovascular disease. The complex findings that make up "metabolic syndrome" include abdominal obesity, high blood pressure, elevated fasting blood sugar, elevated triglycerides and cholesterol, and fatty liver changes. This group of symptoms has also been called "Syndrome X."

These symptoms are *also* abnormalities that can be caused by hypothyroidism. In fact, these patients would have been diagnosed with and treated for hypothyroidism in the days before the TSH test. Instead of recognizing these patients as hypothyroid and treating them accordingly, they are now labeled as having "metabolic syndrome" or "Syndrome X." The proper cure has been hidden because the all-powerful and misleading TSH obscures the appropriate diagnosis.

An ironic result of this laughable yet tragic situation can be found on the consumer website Healthprep.com under the heading "Treating and Managing Metabolic Syndrome."[57] In one paragraph, the writer shares the following wisdom about metabolic syndrome: "Treating the underlying cause is the most important step in preventing, managing, and even reversing metabolic syndrome," followed by this, "the exact causes of metabolic syndrome are unknown." So, the writer is advising the consumer to treat the underlying cause – which of course, is hypothyroidism, but the reader is never told that important little detail – and then the reader is told that the cause is unknown. No wonder there is so much confusion and frustration out there among hypothyroid patients *and* their physicians!

PROPER ROLES IN MEDICAL DECISION MAKING

Remember, medical decision-making often involves analyzing the pros and cons of a proposed intervention in an individual patient. Will a drug or treatment help or hurt a patient? "To treat or not to treat…that is the question," as Hamlet would say. In this day of protocols, guidelines, and best practices, we need to realize that every patient presents with a different set of risk factors, so setting a cutoff that applies to all patients is impossible. Most critical medical decisions present as shades of gray rather than pure black and white. That's why I feel it's so important to make sure that physicians take the time to know as much about each patient as possible and discuss with patients the pros and cons of any proposed treatment.

These days, doctors are often encouraged to let the patient decide which direction she would like to go with her treatment. That's only really appropriate, however, if her doctor first gives her enough information to make these important decisions. Isn't that what *"informed consent"* is all about? If a patient isn't fully informed, it's not genuinely informed consent.

I'm constantly amazed and disappointed when I hear from patients that their gynecologist deferred the decision about whether or not to begin HRT to the patient but did not first give the patient any guidance or data on which to base her decision. Are patients now supposed to be their own physicians? Happily, gone are the days when doctors acted as authoritarians who dictated treatments without any input from patients. But many doctors have gone too far in the opposite direction, handing over all the decision-making responsibility to their patients. I feel strongly that physicians should fully educate their patients first so that the patient can make *educated* decisions. To do otherwise is negligent. The Greek word for doctor, "didaskalos." also means teacher. We should never forget that.

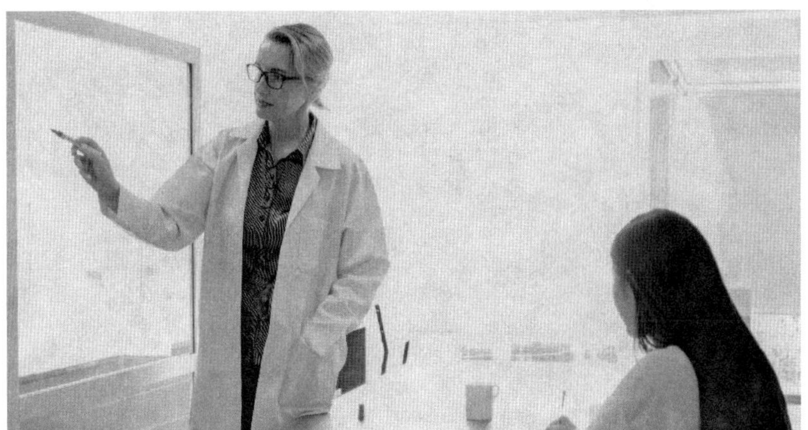

At the same time, I'm not encouraging patients to fully embrace unsourced "advice" online or hastily consult Dr. Google and then march into a doctor's office to demand a particular treatment like they're ordering a burger at a fast-food restaurant. Happily, I've had very few patients try to do this. As a physician, I always tried to the best of my ability to ensure that my patients were well informed and to offer them safe and effective treatments. Then they get to make their properly informed decision about which route they wish to pursue. Hopefully, my training, years of clinical observation, and experience allowed me to do that.

CHAPTER 7: CLINICAL EFFECTS OF WATER RETENTION

"In 1878, Dr. William Ord performed an autopsy on a middle-aged woman who succumbed to hypothyroidism. Upon cutting into her skin, he saw tissues that were thickened and boggy. The tissues appeared to be waterlogged, but no water seeped from his incisions."
~ Mark Starr, MD
from his book "Hypothyroidism, Type 2"

In the past, it was common knowledge that hypothyroidism was a cause of swelling and puffiness, as well as other conditions related to water and fluid retention. It's time that physicians once again reclaim the knowledge of the many ways that lack of thyroid hormone can contribute to these health challenges.

WATER RETENTION, EDEMA

In his 2005 book, *Hypothyroidism Type 2,*[58] pain specialist and ex-chronic pain sufferer Mark Starr, MD, writes extensively about water retention and facial edema (swelling) as classic symptoms of hypothyroidism. I encourage you to read his book because he has done a remarkable job explaining and illustrating this effect. He includes dozens of images of puffy-faced, bloated people before and after proper thyroid replacement. Most of these images were taken from books and articles published in the first half of the 20th century when clinicians knew the significance of puffiness and published their findings.

Nowadays, most clinicians ignore puffiness of the face since we haven't been taught that it has any significance. Instead, facial and undereye puffiness is ignored, considered a part of obesity, or treated as cosmetic problems. And again, there's money to be made. You can drop $260 for a half-ounce of La Mer's "Eye Concentrate." According to La Mer, this "sumptuous cream reduces the appearance of dark circles, lines, and wrinkles."[59] Or, if you want to go the subscription route, order a 2-ounce bottle of "Corrective Eye Serum" – which "targets wrinkles, puffiness"—from "SkinPeutics Cosmeceuticals" auto-delivered every month for $60+ a bottle.[60]

Would it surprise you that compared to pricey eye creams and cosmeceuticals – legally not required to deliver on their marketing claims – the monthly cost for full thyroid hormone replacement can be as little as $5 to $10 a month?

Since the introduction of thyroid blood tests, the medical world appears to have forgotten how to diagnose and treat hypothyroidism and no longer recognizes that undereye and facial puffiness is a classic finding in hypothyroidism. The free market comes to the rescue! "Cosmeceuticals are the new pharmaceuticals" is what happens when the medical community drops the proverbial ball.

CARPAL TUNNEL SYNDROME

Carpal tunnel syndrome can result when water is retained in the tight compartments under the ligaments of the wrist. The median nerve tunnels through the wrist between the wrist's carpal bones on one side and the transverse carpal ligament on the underside of the arm. This tunnel is fairly tight and does not leave much room for changes in the size of the median nerve and its surrounding sheath. This tunnel isn't spared when swelling occurs due to hypothyroidism, particularly in severe hypothyroidism. Consequently, the median nerve becomes pinched. This, in turn, causes varying degrees of pain, tingling, numbness, and weakness in the hand and fingers. This is called carpal tunnel syndrome.

The definitive treatment of carpal tunnel is the surgical "release" – severing – of this tendon. To a casual observer, this seems somewhat barbaric. Why should a perfectly good ligament, part of the normal anatomy, need to be severed? Are the arm and wrist designed so poorly that our normal anatomy needs to be sliced up for us to function properly? Interestingly, surgery was not always the standard of care. But again, we have unlearned so much about hypothyroidism over the years, as the following research illustrates.

A paper by D. N. Golding, presented in 1970 at the Heberden Society meeting in Switzerland,[61] described nine hypothyroid patients who presented with various musculoskeletal symptoms. The author described the case of a 65-year-old woman with hypothyroidism who presented with a two-month history of pain in her forearms and tingling in her hands. The pain was worse in her dominant hand, and she could not hold small objects firmly. She had been diagnosed as hypothyroid five years earlier and put on a small dose of thyroid medication. Doctors gave her a massive 12-fold increase in her dosage of thyroid hormone. (Clearly, they ignored the endocrinology consult here!!!) Her symptoms gradually improved, and when she was seen only four months later, she no longer complained of tingling and clumsiness in her right hand.

The other patients described in this paper also had pain or weakness in other areas. One patient reported much less pain and stiffness, stating that his "joints felt as though they had been oiled with an oil can." Golding said, "In all cases, the symptoms were alleviated by the administration of thyroid hormone." He explained the pathology of this process as follows:

> *"It is now well recognized that paraesthesiae in hypothyroidism usually result from the pressure of oedematous or pseudomucinous material on the median nerves at the wrists causing the carpal tunnel syndrome."*

Fortunately for these nine patients, the prescribing doctor was not afraid to give a high enough dosage of thyroid hormone to make the patients well. Of course, this paper was presented in 1970 when treating hypothyroid patients based on symptomatic response to therapy was still considered reasonable, rather than basing the dose solely on laboratory results. Treating the patient with adequate thyroid hormone reduced the edema, which, in turn, cured the symptoms. No further management was necessary.

Even as late as 1997, we have a report by Perkins and Morgenlander[62] that "hypothyroidism and acromegaly can cause carpal tunnel syndrome and… treatment of the underlying disease is the most successful management approach."

Contrast this simple and effective management plan from 1970 and the paper from 1997 with the more modern approach. A study published just three years later in 2000 by Duyff et al.[63] sought to evaluate neuromuscular signs and symptoms in patients with newly diagnosed hypothyroidism and hyperthyroidism. They found that 79% of the hypothyroid patients had neuromuscular complaints, and a whopping 29% of those studied had carpal tunnel syndrome. "After 1 year of treatment [with enough thyroid to make the TSH normal], 13% of the patients still had weakness…. Weakness in hypothyroidism is more difficult to treat, suggesting myopathy."

Essentially, they are saying that their method of thyroid replacement failed to cure all of the symptoms of carpal tunnel in their hypothyroid patients. Therefore, there must be some other mysterious problem like "neuropathy" that requires some different therapeutic approach. Foolishly, they stopped increasing the thyroid dose as soon as the TSH had normalized, which yielded a suboptimal response. By using the TSH to determine what dose of thyroid to use, they underdosed their patients, which yielded only a partial benefit.

Another paper from the same year by Palumbo et al.[64] studied 26 patients with hypothyroidism who had carpal tunnel syndrome and compared them to 24 healthy controls. They state: "hypothyroidism is commonly included as an important risk factor for carpal tunnel syndrome, yet no study clearly defines the nature of this association." They failed to read Golding's paper from

1970, where he clearly defined this association's exact nature! In this paper, they found that 19 patients (73%) had symptoms of carpal tunnel. "All these symptomatic patients were biochemically euthyroid," which meant their TSH values were normal. The authors concluded that "carpal tunnel syndrome symptoms are common in hypothyroid patients even when they are euthyroid."

Unfortunately for these patients, the fact that they were deemed to be "euthyroid" by lab testing meant that they were not going to be offered thyroid hormone replacement to treat their symptomatic carpal tunnel syndrome. So, what is their option for treatment? Surgery – letting a surgeon sever their transverse carpal ligaments. Indeed, a French study in 2011[65] reported that "there has been a dramatic increase in CTS surgery since the 1990s." That's easy to explain. Modern doctors are no longer treating hypothyroidism adequately due to the widespread adoption of the TSH test. Very sad for hypothyroid patients, but a fabulous business opportunity for the hand surgeon community!

SCALLOPED TONGUE, MACROGLOSSIA

The wrist isn't the only area where edema creates a syndrome or condition. Enter the tongue. "Scalloped tongue" describes a swollen tongue with scalloped edges. The pressure of the teeth against the tongue causes scallop-like indentations in the swollen tissue. (The condition is also sometimes called "pie crust tongue" because the tongue resembles the edges of a pie.) This is similar to when you press your thumb into edematous tissue over your shin if your legs are swollen. The term macroglossia – swollen tongue – is sometimes used to describe the condition. This swelling can also involve the tissues of the soft palate and oropharynx, which can contribute to sleep apnea.

A quick review of the literature over the years shows a similar phenomenon with the evolution, or more accurately the devolution, of the understanding and management of scalloped tongue. In 2006, a study by Jha[66] et al. from Delhi, India, described an association between sleep-disordered breathing (SDB), compromised upper airway, macroglossia, and hypothyroidism.

They studied 50 newly diagnosed, untreated patients with hypothyroidism, did sleep studies on all the patients, and found that 15 (30%) had sleep-disordered breathing at baseline. Of those 15, 12 were treated with "adequate thyroid replacement," and 10 of those (83%) who received *adequate* thyroid got better. In addition, five of these patients also had macroglossia, and four (80%) had complete resolution of the macroglossia with *adequate* thyroid replacement. Sadly, only the abstract of this article is available online, and it does not report what doses of thyroid were considered *"adequate."* But since this study was done in 2006 and not 1970, the doses used were probably based on the normalization of the TSH, which makes the results even more impressive. My guess is that the cure rate would have been closer to 100% if the doctors had been willing to use higher doses.

Finally, in 2018, Melville et al. in Houston[67] published a case study of major macroglossia that developed over 3 months in a patient with myxedema. The patient's tongue had swollen to 16 cm long and 10 cm wide. After the patient had no response to the removal of several suspect medications, a core tongue biopsy was performed. According to the study,

> *"The tissue was positive for Alcian blue and weakly positive for colloidal iron, which are correlated with hypothyroidism and a diagnosis of myxedema. However, the macroglossia did not resolve after correcting for hypothyroidism. The patient required a wedge glossectomy for definitive treatment."*

I can't imagine how awful recovery from a "wedge glossectomy" – removal of part of the tongue – must feel! And while I don't know what dose of thyroid was used in 2018 to "correct" the severe hypothyroidism categorized as "myxedema," my guess is that it was probably not more than 60 to 120 mg (1 to 2 grains) total – only enough was given to make the TSH normal. It's too bad that the patient couldn't have been teleported back to India circa 2006 because Dr. Jha and his team would have given a therapeutic dose of thyroid and given this patient an 80% chance of avoiding a "wedge glossectomy!"

In my practice, I only saw a handful of patients who complained of swollen or thick tongues or who had scalloped tongues. It wasn't a common finding, but it was interesting to see when it was present! But all those who had this problem achieved full resolution of the problem with adequate thyroid replacement. In fact, at one follow-up visit, a patient told me that her scalloped tongue had entirely resolved with her dose, but then, when she ran out of medicine, it came back. When she resumed her therapeutic dose, it resolved again in about 24 hours. The "Amazing Disappearing Scalloped Tongue" sounds like a magic trick! But no magician is needed…just a physician willing to treat a patient until they are well, instead of treating the TSH until it's normal. It's definitely more pleasant than having a "wedge glossectomy," and I'm guessing that patients will prefer it!

SOCK MARKS

Sock marks are the little indentations that occur in edematous legs from the pressure of the elastic at the top of a sock. I remember being taught in medical school that sock marks were signs of two conditions: congestive heart failure or end-stage renal disease. A quick search at MayoClinic.org[68] reveals many other causes of leg swelling. Besides heart failure and related disorders like cardiomyopathy and kidney failure, other causes include chemotherapy, cirrhosis, deep vein thrombosis and thrombophlebitis, hormone therapy, lymphedema, obesity, pain relievers, pregnancy, prescription medications, pulmonary hypertension, sitting for a long time, standing for a long time, venous insufficiency, rheumatoid arthritis, osteoarthritis, and of course various injuries to the lower extremities such as a broken ankle or a burn. Amazingly, hypothyroidism is *never* mentioned on the Mayo Clinic's list!!!

Isn't it fascinating that we know so much about swelling in the legs but also so little? Although I didn't keep strict records about the frequency of seeing sock marks, it was a very common finding in my hypothyroid patients – and far more common than a scalloped tongue. But like scalloped tongue and carpal tunnel syndrome, it is almost always resolved entirely with adequate thyroid replacement.

When a hypothyroid patient has the return of carpal tunnel, scalloped tongue, or sock marks, this is a sign that a dosage adjustment is needed. What is challenging is determining whether that swelling suggests underdose or overdose because both can trigger the issue.

If the thyroid dose is too high, it elevates the resting pulse, which causes the heart to beat less efficiently. Think about gas mileage when you drive your car too fast. Your vehicle uses fuel more efficiently at 55 miles per hour than at 75 miles per hour. It's the same for your heart. An elevated resting heart rate can cause a mild and transient form of heart failure – pump failure – which disrupts and obstructs the smooth flow of blood, which in turn causes swelling in the tissues. This can also be accompanied by mild shortness of breath or new exercise intolerance, again due to inefficiency of cardiac function. The solution is to lower the dose of thyroid hormone.

So, when there are swelling-related symptoms, and it's not clear whether the dose was a bit too high or low, the simplest way to figure it out was to lower the dose – or better yet, stop for a few days – and see if the swelling gets better or worse. If it resolves, the dose is too high. If the swelling worsens, the dose is too low, and now it's even more inadequate. If that case, increase the dose to the point where swelling goes away, but not enough to cause any symptoms of overmedication.

MYXEDEMA AND MYXEDEMA COMA

Water retention isn't restricted to just the face. Women with hypothyroidism can also retain water in other parts of their bodies. Fingers get puffy, rings get tight, and ankles and feet get swollen, particularly later in the day. What causes this puffiness? The following passage from Dr. Mark Starr's excellent book, *Hypothyroidism: Type 2,* explains how myxedema is, as Dr. Starr states, a "telltale sign of hypothyroidism:"

> *In 1878, Dr. William Ord performed an autopsy on a middle-aged woman who succumbed to hypothyroidism. Upon cutting*

into her skin, he saw tissues that were thickened and boggy. The tissues appeared to be waterlogged, but no water seeped from his incisions. Dr. Ord realized this disease was unique and previously unrecognized.

Dr. Ord summoned a leading chemist named Halleburton to help identify the substance causing the swelling. What they found was an abnormally large accumulation of mucin. Mucin is a normal constituent of our tissues. It is a jelly-like material that spontaneously accumulated in hypothyroidism. Mucin grabs onto water and causes swelling. Dr. Halleburton found 50 times the normal amount of mucin in the woman's skin. Her other tissues also contained excess mucin.

The doctors coined the term 'myxedema.' 'Myx' is the Greek word for mucin, and 'edema' means swelling. 'Myxedema' was adopted as the medical term for severe hypothyroidism."

The term "myxedema" isn't commonly used to describe hypothyroidism, but I remember learning about "myxedema coma" back in medical school. Myxedema coma is the often-fatal end stage of long-standing untreated hypothyroidism. A 1955 article by VK Summers, MD in Liverpool,[69] describes four individual cases of myxedema coma, and all were fatal. The ages of the patients ranged from 59 to 65, and each presented with a puffy face, pale, dry skin, slowed mental function, croaking voice, very low body temperature, low and weak pulse, and drowsiness that proceeded within a few days to coma, and eventual death. Each was treated with thyroid replacement orally and by subcutaneous injections, but apparently, it was too little and too late for these four individuals.

A similar case study report from Spain was published in 2019,[70] reporting on four patients ranging from 67 to 86 with similar presentations. Fortunately, in this report, three out of four patients survived after aggressive intravenous thyroid hormone replacement. Happily, over these past 60+ years, we have learned that giving thyroid hormone intravenously works better than the oral or subcutaneous route in severely hypothyroid patients who are sliding into a myxedema coma. That's good to know, but it's far better to prevent it entirely by fully replacing thyroid long before a patient is anywhere near this dangerous state.

HOARSENESS

Our ability to speak and sing is also affected by hypothyroidism. Though it's not a universal symptom, hoarseness of the voice isn't uncommon and is considered a classic symptom of hypothyroidism. Though many general articles about hypothyroidism list hoarseness as one of the common presenting symptoms, it's difficult to find a mention of hypothyroidism if one searches the literature for articles on "causes of hoarseness." For example, a German article from 1995 by Muller[71] lists the following as possible causes of hoarseness: "functional disorders of the voice, inflammation of the larynx, secondary changes of the vocal folds, polyps, cysts, edema, papillomas, tumors, trauma, or palsies of the vocal cords due to different reasons."

A 2009 study by Schwartz, Cohen, and Dailey et al.[72] adds the following possible causes to the list:

> *"Recent surgical procedures involving the neck or affecting the recurrent laryngeal nerve, recent endotracheal intubation, radiation treatment to the neck a history of tobacco abuse, and occupation as a singer or vocal performer."*

I couldn't find "endocrine abnormalities" or "thyroid dysfunction" listed as a cause of hoarseness anywhere. The treatments for hoarseness in these studies included anti-reflux medication, voice therapy, voice rest, vocal hygiene, and surgery for anatomic lesions. There was no mention of thyroid replacement. A German study from 2015 by Reiter, Hoffmann, et al.[73] imperiously proclaimed that "the *only* entity causing hoarseness that can be treated pharmacologically is chronic laryngitis associated with gastro-esophageal reflux, which responds to treatment of the reflux disorder."

Well, I guess the science is settled! (At least it seems to be in Germany!)

What's bypassed the standard medical wisdom in Germany and elsewhere is that the quality of the voice is affected by several hormones, including thyroid, estrogen, and testosterone. We've all heard older women with deep, husky, hoarse voices. (Think Bea Arthur, who played Maude and starred in Golden Girls.) In my opinion, when an older woman's voice becomes deep or hoarse, it's likely to be a sign of hormonal imbalance. I strongly suspect many of these women are postmenopausal, still have ovaries, and don't take estrogen replacement. As a gynecologist, I saw in action how the pitch of the voice depends on the balance of estrogen vs. testosterone. When estrogen is plentiful, as it is when women are young, the voice is higher-pitched and girlish. But later, when estrogen production declines, testosterone becomes dominant, and the voice will deepen (sometimes accompanied by the much-dreaded appearance of chin hairs!)

The physiologic cause of this is as follows: As the ovaries lose their function, the first thing that goes is the ability to ovulate and to make progesterone. The next function to go is the ability to produce estrogen, and finally, usually years later, testosterone production declines. So, hoarseness is often a sign that a woman is in that phase of life where her ovaries and adrenal glands are still making testosterone, but estrogen production is severely diminished. Thus, the voice becomes more manly after menopause, particularly if women mistakenly choose not to replace their estrogen starting at the onset of menopause.

Thyroid deficiency typically makes the voice hoarser rather than deep – but sometimes, the voice has both qualities. I suspect this is due to polysaccharide infiltration of the vocal cords, edema, or possibly sluggishness of the muscles involved. Whatever the cause, I argue that, based on my experience, hoarseness is one of the most manageable symptoms of hypothyroidism to reverse with thyroid replacement. The literature confirms my experience. A 2003 Chinese study by Zhibin Wang[74] evaluated 32 patients with "throat symptoms," including hoarseness, who were treated with thyroid replacement. The thyroid symptoms disappeared in 27 and improved in 5. All the patients studied were improved or cured with thyroid. That's an incredible response rate.

Several of my patients were paid to use their voices. I worked with several patients who were voice instructors or coaches and several professional opera singers. One of those is quite famous and can be seen from time to time on TV and stage at the Kennedy Center and the Metropolitan Opera House. After we addressed their hypothyroidism, they all had significantly improved singing voices. Perhaps thyroid replacement has even prolonged a few careers along the way! What an easy cure and a fantastic result!

CHAPTER 8: SKIN AND HAIR

"Hair brings one's self-image into focus; it is vanity's proving ground. Hair is terribly personal, a tangle of mysterious prejudices."
~Shana Alexander

The health of skin and hair is directly related to the availability and function of thyroid hormone. Still, women spend countless amounts of money searching for remedies for dry skin and hair loss when there's an easy, inexpensive solution. Let's examine the connection between skin, hair, and thyroid hormones.

SKIN CONDITIONS, DRYNESS

Besides the almost universal finding of dry, often itchy skin, the skin provides many other hypothyroidism clues. Eczema is a relatively common condition affecting the hands, arms, face, and upper eyelids; it typically improves with adequate replacement. In the winter, some women develop painful vertical cracks or cuts in the fingertips. Many hypothyroid patients report symmetrical patches of small bumps on the backs of their upper arms. This condition is called keratosis pilaris, and it's caused by proteinaceous material clogging the hair follicles. An itchy, burning scalp is also very common in hypothyroid patients. The nails are also often affected and are usually thin, brittle, flaking, cracking, and vertically ridged. I found that all of these skin and nail conditions resolve with full thyroid replacement.

Vitiligo – white patches of skin that lose their natural melanin and color – is three times more common in hypothyroid patients than normal[75] and can regress somewhat with thyroid (though a complete cure is unlikely.)

Infections of the skin are also more common in hypothyroid patients. Fungal infections like tinea, yeast infections in the skin folds, folliculitis, and acne can improve significantly with thyroid replacement. Nail fungus can often be found on the toenails of hypothyroid patients, particularly when the feet are icy. It can clear up if you replace enough thyroid to make the feet consistently warm.

Hives – also known as urticaria – are a relatively rare finding in hypothyroidism and are usually present only in the most severe cases. Proper thyroid dosing can cure them. And just to keep you on your toes, thyroid replacement can sometimes cause hives. So, pay attention to hives to see whether they improve or get worse as the dose of thyroid hormone is adjusted.

Dry eyes are also quite common with hypothyroidism and usually respond nicely to thyroid replacement to the extent that patients can stop using moisturizing eyedrops multiple times a day. Similarly, dryness of the mouth is also occasionally seen, though not nearly as common, and it improves as well. (The patient's dentist will appreciate this.) An association between hypothyroidism and Sjogren's Syndrome – which can cause severe dry eye and mouth symptoms – has been known for years. In 2007, Luis Jara, Carmen Navarro, et al. reported the following[76]:

> *"The coexistence of pSS [primary Sjogren's syndrome] and thyroiditis is frequent and suggests a common genetic or environmental factor predisposition with similar pathogenic mechanisms. PSS was ten times more frequent in patients with autoimmune thyroid disease and autoimmune thyroiditis was nine times more frequent in pSS."*

In patients with Sjogren's Syndrome, the condition is likely to improve somewhat and may completely resolve with proper thyroid replacement.

When the patient presents with significant skin symptoms, I have learned that giving at least some natural desiccated thyroid is usually a good idea. The epithelium – the skin, etc. covering our body surfaces – seems particularly sensitive to T3. But keep in mind that too much T3 can cause acne or oiliness of the skin. The goal is enough T3 to make the skin normal, but not so much to make it baby soft or oily.

HAIR LOSS

Hair loss is one of the most common – and often one of the most frustrating and demoralizing – symptoms of hypothyroidism and one that brought many patients in to see me. Hair loss was the symptom that made *me* start asking questions and eventually start taking thyroid hormone! Women do not like losing their hair!

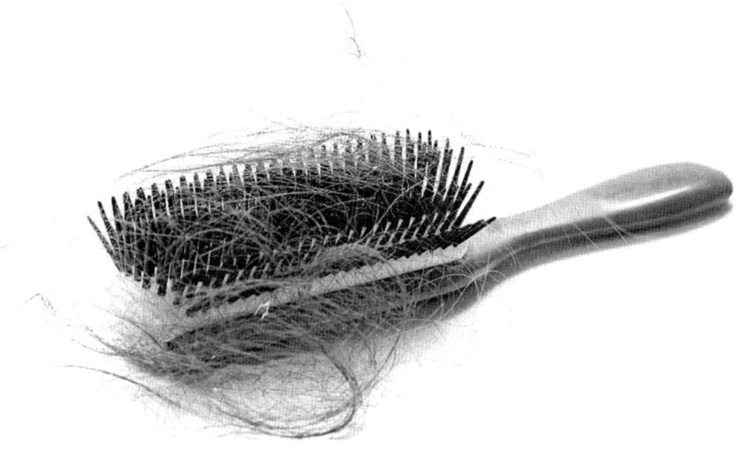

If the metabolic rate is low because thyroid function is inadequate, not enough heat is produced in the body. Essentially, there aren't enough logs on the internal fire. Instead, the calories consumed when the patient is hypothyroid are stored as fat instead of being turned into heat or energy. When the body is cold, it tries to conserve heat by redirecting warm blood flow away from the extremities. Consequently, the hands, feet, and legs are cold to the touch, and I suspect that blood is also redirected away from the scalp. Nails are usually not healthy when hands and feet are cold, so how can hair be healthy if there is no blood flow to the scalp?

(Hint: it can't!) Hair that grows on a scalp with insufficient blood flow will become thin and fragile and often fall out or break off.

When I started taking thyroid myself more than 20 years ago, I had been losing quite a bit of hair for some time. After starting a dose of about 3 grains of Thyrolar (a synthetic T4/T3 version of natural desiccated thyroid that is no longer available) in a split dose, my hair stopped falling out. It started growing back in about three weeks!

I've found that fixing hair loss with thyroid can sometimes be simple, but sometimes it's not as easy as we'd like. I usually started with some natural desiccated thyroid since hair, like skin, also seems to want some T3, but I recommend being careful with it. It's not uncommon for hair loss to recur with too much T3. Even more interestingly, hair loss sometimes returns after a patient has been stable on a dose of natural desiccated thyroid for a few years. In that case, I partly or entirely removed the natural desiccated thyroid and gave a T4 product to make the hair happy again. That's what happened to me. Now, 20 years later, I am currently on just T4, and my hair is fine. If I take even a tiny amount of natural desiccated thyroid (containing T3), or if I take too much or too little T4, my hair loss recurs.

So, I advise paying close attention to hair loss in case it recurs after optimized thyroid treatment. If it does recur, assuming other symptoms of overdose or underdose aren't present, the best approach is to replace some or all of the natural desiccated thyroid with an equal amount of straight T4. My theory is that the T3 in natural desiccated thyroid may be accumulating in the tissues over time and can eventually begin to cause hair loss that it had previously resolved. I also have noticed that many hypothyroid patients need less T3 after many years of taking it. Why does this happen? I don't know. But I've seen it happen many times, though it's not a universal phenomenon. But I recommend watching for it, especially for women who are on only natural desiccated thyroid with no added T4.

CHAPTER 9: SLUGGISH GASTROINTESTINAL TRACT

"Thyroid disease is common, and its effects on the gastrointestinal system are protean…
The gastrointestinal manifestations of thyroid disease are generally due to reduced motility in hypothyroidism…Symptoms usually resolve with treatment of the thyroid disease."
~ EC Ebert[77]

Let's look at the many effects thyroid hormone has on the digestive tract. You may be amazed how many common gastrointestinal symptoms are, in fact, related to thyroid deficiency – and how easily they can be resolved.

ANOREXIA, GASTROPARESIS

First, it's important to understand that the gastrointestinal (GI) tract allows us to nourish ourselves by absorbing calories and nutrients from our food. To accomplish that vital function, we need to take food in, break it down into small pieces, digest the food, absorb the nutrients we need, and eliminate what we don't need. It seems simple enough, but in the absence of adequate thyroid function, many conditions can disrupt this process.

Peristalsis is the term we use to describe the synchronized, worm-like squeezing action of the layer of smooth muscle that encircles our esophagus and intestines and gradually pushes food through the alimentary canal. It functions like "the wave" in a stadium, gradually pushing the contents of our GI tract from one end to the other. When thyroid hormone function is inadequate, this peristalsis is slowed down to varying degrees. Gastroparesis is the fancy medical term that describes a severe form of this condition. In essence, gastroparesis means that the force that normally pushes the contents of the GI tract downward is weak. The squeezing muscles are sluggish.

The lack of this forward movement in the GI tract, due to lack of adequate stimulation by thyroid hormone, will cause any number of conditions – all the same problem affecting different areas of the GI tract. Pustorino, Foti, Calipari, et al.[78] discuss this in an Italian paper published in 2004. They state that "thyroid diseases may be related to symptoms due to digestive motility dysfunction…Any segment of the gastrointestinal tract may be involved."

Starting from the top of the GI tract, the first condition caused by this gut sluggishness is simply a lack of appetite, also known as anorexia. This isn't the kind of anorexia seen in young girls and women who have a distorted body image and see themselves as obese when they are anything but, and purposely want to make themselves skinnier than they already are. Instead, this medical term describes a person who is not hungry. When they force themselves to eat something, they feel full quickly, after only a few bites. These women often deny that they have a small appetite because they eat until they are full, but if you ask them specifically how much food they eat compared to what their friends eat, they'll often admit that they eat less. They may skip meals because they simply forget to eat and are never hungry.

While not trying to lose weight, these women are often quite thin because their GI tracts are simply not working, and they end up calorie and nutrient deficient. They will also often be anemic due to deficiencies of iron and other nutrients. I'll never forget my young 12-year-old patient Jenna, who was brought to see me by her mom, a drug representative who knew I treated thyroid problems. We briefly mentioned her earlier when we discussed the bone effects of hypothyroidism. Jenna weighed only 64 pounds at the age of 12. She looked like a child, not an adolescent. During her first visit, she kept her head on my desk because she was too tired to hold it up for the duration of the visit. She admitted that she was never hungry and got full very easily. Her hands felt like little popsicles. Her morning temperature was consistently well under 97 degrees.

The sad part of this story is that this sweet young lady had already had several endoscopies – and even a few colonoscopies – as her doctors attempted to identify her particular GI malady. After multiple invasive procedures, doctors concluded that Jenna had "gastroparesis" and sent her on her way without any treatment for her condition. Welcome to modern medicine. Apparently, all these gastroenterologists had never been taught that thyroid hormone drives peristalsis. They failed to make that crucial link.

As I suspected in this thin, waiflike little girl, her bone density was very low for her age, which was to be expected given her mild involuntary starvation. I have seen this be true not infrequently in thin, petite women who also have icy hands and get full after two bites of food. They almost all have very low bone mass. Happily, this situation is easy to reverse with thyroid replacement. This is particularly interesting because most people with casual knowledge of thyroid fear its use. After all, it's supposed to cause bone loss. (And when overmedicated with thyroid hormone, that is certainly true.) But in these women, thyroid hormone can be beneficial!

In this case, it only took 75 mcg of levothyroxine to wake up Jenna's GI tract and make her well. Within the next 14 months, she gained 26 pounds, grew 4 inches, and her bone density in her spine increased 21%! Amazing! And all it took was enough thyroid to stimulate peristalsis and get her GI tract functional again! Her mom told me at the follow-up visit that for the first time in Jenna's life, she had asked for a snack when she came home from school! She blossomed into a young woman in front of our eyes after this tiny dose of thyroid restored her appetite! What a fabulous response!

SWALLOWING DISORDERS

When hypothyroidism disrupts peristalsis, patients often complain of feeling like they aren't able to swallow food or drink properly, and that food "gets stuck" in their esophagus. This is called *dysphagia*, or an *esophageal motility disorder*. This swallowing dysfunction can be documented by different radiologic and endoscopic procedures, none of which are particularly pleasant.

If you visit the Mayo Clinic's discussion of dysphagia online,[79] you will see that the recommended treatments for dysphagia include swallowing exercises, esophageal dilatation, liquid diets, feeding tubes, cutting the muscle that encircles the bottom of the esophagus via a laparoscope, placing a stent in the esophagus, etc. There is no mention of hypothyroidism as a cause of this problem or thyroid hormone replacement as a treatment.

However, a cursory review of the medical literature reveals a Brazilian Portuguese study published in 2017[80] that showed a 66.7% prevalence of swallowing complaints among patients with thyroid disease. Further, case reports published in 1982 by Eastwood et al.[81] and in 2001 by Urquhart et al.[82] describe individual patients with severe hypothyroidism who also had severe esophageal motility disorders. In both cases, their esophageal conditions were *entirely* resolved with proper thyroid hormone replacement.

This knowledge proves very helpful because, in the elderly, an inability to swallow can lead to life-threatening aspiration pneumonia. Curing dysphagia with thyroid hormone in these patients can prevent them from choking on food and developing aspiration pneumonia.

In addition, a 2014 study by Ilhan et al.[83] found a statistically significant increased prevalence of esophageal muscle abnormalities in hypothyroid patients compared to normal controls. Those authors note that the "Gastrointestinal tract is one of the most affected systems in hypothyroidism." Unfortunately, the gastroenterologists who typically treat these conditions don't know that. But then, if they did, all those lucrative procedures wouldn't be so necessary.

REFLUX, GERD

The terms dyspepsia, gastroesophageal reflux disease (GERD), acid reflux, and heartburn all refer to the inability of the stomach to empty itself efficiently. Again, this is a function of peristalsis not working correctly at the stomach level. These patients are often on histamine-2 blockers or proton pump inhibitor drugs like Pepcid and Nexium to reduce acid production. As we know, by decreasing acid production, these drugs can also block the ability of the stomach to digest food, thus causing certain nutritional deficiencies. These drugs also cause many other side effects, so if they can be avoided, they should. But the only way to avoid those drugs is to fix the underlying problem with peristalsis. And how do we encourage the stomach to empty itself properly? You guessed it: add thyroid hormone.

I found that giving enough thyroid to patients with GERD allowed them to eliminate their daily dependence on these drugs and over-the-counter antacids like TUMS. And, since they were no longer blocking acid production with drugs, these patients regained the ability to digest food properly and absorb the nutrients therein.

One way to tell that nutrient absorption is improved in this situation is that bone density will often improve, as I saw in the young girl with gastroparesis. Similarly, conditions like iron deficiency anemia will also resolve with time. Win, win! Funny how things get better when you just get the body working again by replacing missing hormones!

ABDOMINAL BLOATING AND DISTENSION

As we proceed down the GI tract, the next problems we see from sluggish peristalsis are bloating and abdominal distension. This symptom tends to get worse after eating and later in the day. These women complain of an expanding waistline, even without any weight gain. Clothes feel tight, and these women feel uncomfortable. What's happening is that the intestines aren't doing what they're supposed to, which is to gradually squeeze/push the digesting food downward towards the colon so the nutrients can be absorbed, and waste can eventually be excreted. Instead, the hypothyroid intestine is very lazy. The smooth muscle wall isn't contracting, and the intestines become distended and swollen. Consequently, the entire abdomen also becomes swollen and distended.

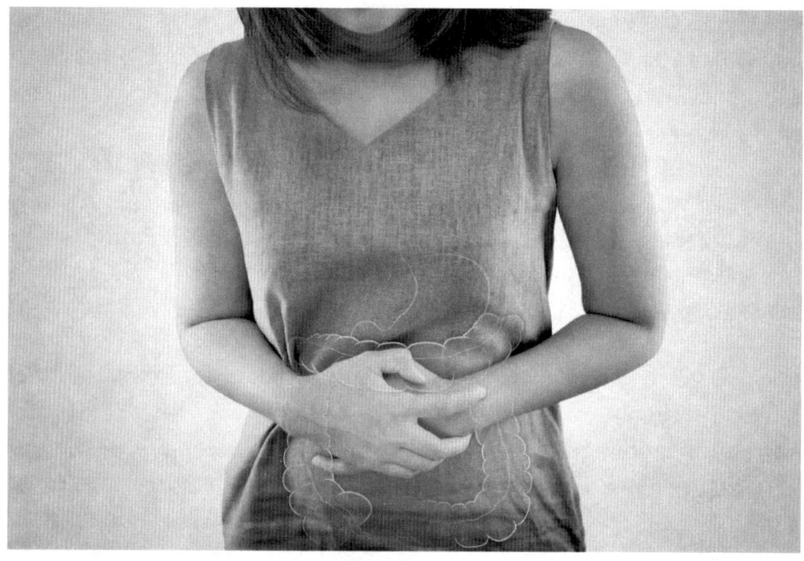

A 1990 article from a Croatian team of researchers[84] describes a 64-year-old woman with hypothyroidism and intestinal pseudo-obstruction. They wrote:

> *"Characteristic intestinal hypomotility in severe hypothyroidism may progress to intestinal pseudo-obstruction, paralytic ileus and megacolon. These rare but potentially serious complications must be recognized and treated promptly with adequate doses of thyroid hormone replacement therapy."*

In 1996, an Italian study by Fiorani et al.[85] described a 71-year-old woman with megacolon and other symptoms of severe hypothyroidism, including drowsiness and shortness of breath. They found that:

> *"Treatment with levothyroxine caused a progressive improvement of the general condition of the patient and of the megacolon so that the authors hypothesize that the intestinal pseudo-obstruction was caused by the hypothyroidism."*

One might wonder if something in the Adriatic Sea is toxic to thyroid glands!

On a side note, it's interesting that in the Italian study, the authors suggest that combining T3 and T4 is preferable to only using T4 when treating patients with such a severe presentation. I have found that to be true as well. Specifically, after treating many hypothyroid patients with sluggish bowels, it has been my impression that bowel dysfunction is *very* sensitive to T3. I believe that all smooth and striated muscle is particularly sensitive to T3. So, in most cases, when patients present with symptoms suggesting a sluggish GI tract, I usually include at least some natural desiccated thyroid or T3 in their therapeutic regimen.

The result of adding thyroid to this sluggish GI tract is that as smooth muscle tone is increased and the intestines tighten up to their normal size, they are no longer distended and flaccid, and the rhythmic, synchronized contractions of peristalsis are restored to normal. This is why the distension disappears, and things start moving again.

A study of GI transit time published in 1984 by Shafer et al.[86] confirmed this result. In this study, the authors fed hypothyroid patients a nonabsorbable carbohydrate and measured how fast it traveled through the GI tract with and without thyroid replacement. As one would expect, they found that "Transit time decreased significantly when hypothyroid patients were given thyroid replacement (p less than 0.01)." Of course, none of this is surprising if one understands gut physiology and peristalsis and what drives it.

SIBO, MALNUTRITION

SIBO stands for Small Intestine Bacterial Overgrowth – a condition where the gut has an unhealthy balance of bacteria.

Recently, SIBO has been a bit of a trendy diagnosis in integrative, alternative, anti-aging, and nutritional medicine. The treatments offered for SIBO are usually complex. They sometimes include antibiotics, various dietary restrictions, and many expensive supplements (often sold directly to the patient by the practitioner. Hmmm.) A quick internet search reveals that the specific cause of SIBO is elusive. In my opinion, that often means that we're not dealing with a distinct disease but rather with a symptom of something else that has not yet been identified. Some of the many causes of SIBO listed online include low stomach acid, pre-existing medical conditions such as diabetes and lupus, gluten, alcohol, refined sugar, over-the-counter medications, gut dysmotility, and decreased transit time within the small bowel.

There you have it. Gut dysmotility and decreased transit time, which can be caused by hypothyroidism, will cause the flow of bowel contents to slow down, even allowing some retrograde flow. That, in turn, will enable bacteria that belong in the large bowel to travel upstream and set up shop in the small intestine. This led me to conclude that SIBO isn't a disease in itself. Instead, it's yet another consequence of the widespread disruption of normal bodily functions that occurs with reduced thyroid function. I think treatment for SIBO should start with thyroid replacement, and we can leave the expensive supplements on the practitioner's shelf.

There's another aspect of the sluggishness of the hypothyroid bowel and the bacterial overgrowth caused by bacteria floating upstream. I have found that patients with a sluggish gut, low appetite, bloating, etc., are often nutritionally deficient because the gut can't absorb nutrients effectively. They are usually low on Vitamin D and often iron deficient as well. We would likely find other deficiencies if more comprehensive nutrient testing were done. It's not uncommon to find that these patients have been eating a limited and sometimes reduced-calorie diet for years, limiting the number of nutrients available to be absorbed.

There's another issue as well. The GI tract is lined with villi whose job is to "suck" in nutrients and send them into the bloodstream and the lymphatic system. These villi become lazy and sluggish and aren't effective at absorbing nutrients. So, the patient fails to absorb the few nutrients they have eaten. So even if the patient is eating a nutrient-rich diet, she can still end up malnourished.

One of the easiest ways to assess the long-term overall nutritional status of someone with reduced nutrient absorption is to do a bone density test. Women who have not been digesting and absorbing their nutrients for years tend to have quite low bone density because you can't make bone if you don't have the required building blocks. And without a well-functioning gut, there aren't enough nutrients available to build dense bones, even if estrogen is adequate.

In addition, those same nutrient deficiencies are likely to create other problems with the immune system, for example, since you can't make immune cells and antibodies without certain nutrients. Consequently, it's crucial to get the gut of a hypothyroid patient working again, so the rest of the patient's body can get the nutrients needed for all those functions to work correctly.

Once the thyroid deficiency is resolved with the proper amount of replacement, we can expect excellent bone density growth due to the improved flow of nutrients into the body now that the gut is functioning again. It's fun to watch and sound proof that we're on the right track!

CONSTIPATION

According to the famous Irish writer, poet, and playwright Samuel Beckett, "Constipation is a sign of good health in Pomeranians." I'm not sure why he said that about fluffy little dogs, but it's the exact *opposite* in humans. Constipation is a sign of bad health in humans. It's also a common sign of poor thyroid function. My experience with this problem was quite personal and longstanding until I started taking thyroid replacement in 1998. Looking back, I now realize that before I began taking thyroid hormone, I did not even know that a normal unstrained bowel movement was possible! After just three days on thyroid hormone, my own bathroom experience was transformed! Indeed, complete resolution of chronic constipation is one of the *easiest* goals to achieve with thyroid replacement. In my experience, we just need to ensure that a constipated patient gets the necessary thyroid hormone dose – and the problem is solved!

Constipation is the apparent consequence of decreased peristalsis affecting the colon. Because hypothyroidism allows the waste material to sit in the colon for a longer time instead of being pushed along via peristalsis, the contents become increasingly dehydrated and hardened. This, in turn, makes elimination more difficult. Since thyroid replacement decreases transit time, the stool passes through more quickly and can be easily eliminated before dehydrating and hardening.

Another issue is that taking too much thyroid hormone – especially when it includes T3 – may cause diarrhea. What was very interesting to me is that this can creep up after years of being stable on a particular dose.

I saw this in several patients over the years. Each was on full thyroid hormone replacement, taking NDT for several years, and then developed unexplained diarrhea. None of them thought to mention it to me and instead consulted with their gastroenterologists and ended up with workups that would reveal no specific cause. One patient's problem was so severe that she had bowel accidents! These women were prescribed various medications to treat the symptoms of diarrhea. When I received consultation notes from those gastroenterologists, I would immediately call these patients to get more information about what transpired. The symptoms usually developed slowly and worsened until they finally sought medical help.

I reminded them that diarrhea is listed as a possible side effect of thyroid on the list of overdose symptoms I hand out at the start of thyroid treatment. And then I always asked, "Why didn't you call me when you first developed diarrhea?" The answer was always the same: "I've been ok on this dose for so long that I didn't think it had anything to do with my thyroid dose."

I would then explain that overdose effects can happen *at any time*, which is why patients need to remain vigilant in watching for those symptoms weeks, months, and years after starting thyroid treatment.

As I mentioned before, I suspect that seeing this symptom develop years after starting treatment is due to T3's proclivity to be stored in the tissues to the point of excess. When there is too much T3, peristalsis speeds up excessively, and diarrhea ensues. The best way to remove the excess T3 effect is to stop the intake of any thyroid. I had these patients stop their thyroid medication and call me back in a week. In every case, diarrhea stopped within a week. But typically, the women again had signs and symptoms of hypothyroidism soon after that. The first symptoms were usually those related to lack of T4 – fatigue and feeling cold. At that point, I would add back some thyroid, generally starting with just T4. I only added T3 much later if needed to achieve full wellness.

Another problem with thyroid overdose is, believe it or not, the resumption of constipation! I'm not sure why this happens in certain patients, but I suspect it's due to excessive tone in the smooth muscle in the bowel wall that gently squeezes the colon *too* tightly, causing a mild mechanical obstruction. The result of this is constipation. And just like diarrhea, the treatment is to withhold all supplemental thyroid until this constipation resolves.

The bottom line is that constipation can be present with too little thyroid and too much thyroid. So, you need to pay close attention to see if there are any other symptoms of overdose or underdose present, and you also need to assess how this symptom changes as the dosage changes. If constipation is getting better, you're going in the right direction with the dose, and if it's getting worse, you need to go in the other direction. Simple. Remember that constipation can occur at both ends of the thyroid spectrum.

CHAPTER 10: LIVER DISORDERS

"Save the liver!"
~ Dan Aykroyd, portraying Julia Child in the Saturday Night Live skit "The French Chef" in 1978

The liver is an essential organ that helps with digestion, metabolism, detoxification, filtering toxins from the bloodstream, synthesizing protein, and storing vitamins and minerals. And, like every other organ in the human body, the liver takes orders from the thyroid gland. When there's insufficient thyroid hormone, all the liver's various functions can suffer, as I review in this chapter.

"SAVE THE LIVER!"

Rohit Sinha, Brijesh Singh, and Paul Yen, from their labs in Singapore and India,[87] recently published a comprehensive review of the literature on the effects of thyroid hormone on the liver. They state the following:

> *"It has been known for a long time that thyroid hormones have prominent effects on hepatic fatty acid and cholesterol synthesis and metabolism. Indeed, hypothyroidism has been associated with increased serum levels of triglycerides and cholesterol as well as non-alcoholic fatty liver disease (NAFLD)...Thyroid hormone mediates these effects at the transcriptional and post-translational levels and via autophagy. Given these potentially beneficial effects on lipid metabolism, it is possible that thyroid*

> *hormone analogues and / or mimetics might be useful for the treatment of metabolic disease involving the liver, such as hypercholesterolaemia and NAFLD.*
>
> *In mammals, thyroid hormones are critical regulators of metabolism, development and growth. Many of the metabolic activities regulated by thyroid hormones are related to the anabolism and/or catabolism of macromolecules that affect energy homeostasis during different nutritional conditions, such as proteins, lipids and carbohydrates."*

In slightly simpler words, when thyroid function is too low, the cholesterol is high, and when thyroid function is excessive, as in hyperthyroidism, cholesterol is abnormally low. It's the same for triglycerides. This is a very predictable and dose-related effect. The worse the hypothyroidism, the higher the cholesterol tends to be. In addition, thyroid affects other metabolic functions by controlling the synthesis of proteins in the cells.

LIVER MALFUNCTION

As I discussed earlier, over half a century ago, the association between hypothyroidism and elevated cholesterol was well known. Measurement of cholesterol in the blood was even used to confirm the clinical diagnosis of hypothyroidism. But this association has not been taught to medical students for many decades, so most modern doctors aren't aware of it. As a result, high cholesterol is viewed as a disease unto itself and not just a manifestation of impaired thyroid function. This means that the approach to treating high cholesterol has sadly revolved around "lifestyle changes" and drugs that directly lower cholesterol instead of addressing the underlying thyroid hormone deficiency causing the cholesterol to be elevated. What else is new, right? Diagnosing and treating the underlying cause of conditions is never the approach of modern medicine anymore. That would challenge the modern philosophy that every symptom needs a drug, making way too much sense!

"A healthy lifestyle is the first defense against high cholesterol. But sometimes diet and exercise aren't enough, and you might need to take cholesterol medications," we are advised by the Mayo Clinic Staff at MayoClinic.org.[88] Indeed, we have all been taught to place the blame for high cholesterol directly at the feet of the patient! They're eating the wrong foods, not exercising enough, or they foolishly chose the wrong parents who passed along a genetic tendency to have high cholesterol. Then, we make a patient feel like a failure when her efforts to "eat better and exercise more" fail. (And, of course, they almost always fail because diet and exercise aren't the main determinants of cholesterol level.) After that, we start prescribing statins, bile sequestrants, or fibrate drugs to force the cholesterol down. Astonishingly, thyroid is no longer even mentioned in current lists of medications that lower cholesterol.

Some of these drugs work well, some don't, and many have potentially severe side effects. I had a patient whose uncle died of a complication from a statin drug. Yikes! Myositis – muscle pain secondary to inflammation of the muscles – is one of the most frequent adverse effects of popular statin drugs. The other big concern with statin drugs is their potentially damaging effect on the liver. For years, doctors were advised to regularly check "liver function" tests in patients on statins to screen for liver damage.

Other side effects listed by Web MD[89] include diarrhea, constipation, nausea, abdominal cramps, vomiting, headache, dizziness, drowsiness, fatigue, difficulty sleeping, and rash or flushed skin. None of these side effects of these cholesterol-lowering drugs seem particularly desirable. I'll rely on thyroid replacement to normalize cholesterol values in my patients, thank you very much!

My experience with starting thyroid replacement is a perfect example of this effect. When I began taking thyroid 20 some years ago, I went to a gym regularly and was relatively slender and fit, eating a primarily vegetarian, clean diet. Yet my total cholesterol was in the 210 to 220 range. It was not at all fair as far as I was concerned. But then, at that time, I was also chronically constipated, freezing cold, tired, and shedding hair like crazy. After reading Broda Barnes' book and finding my therapeutic dose of thyroid, my repeat cholesterol level was 160. Nowadays, several decades later, I eat bacon regularly, don't exercise as much as I did back then, and picked up a few pounds along the way, and my cholesterol remains at 165.

So contrary to the opinion of the experts at the much-lauded Mayo Clinic, my prior "healthy lifestyle" seemed to have had a negligible effect on my cholesterol compared to the dramatic benefits of adequately replacing thyroid hormone. Further, I have seen similarly impressive reductions in cholesterol levels in many of my patients. I've come to expect that cholesterol levels usually end up in the 160 to 170 range in most patients on optimal thyroid replacement. Only a handful of patients needed statin drugs, which makes me very happy. Perhaps I should send the Mayo Clinic a note about this little secret that was common knowledge 65 years ago!

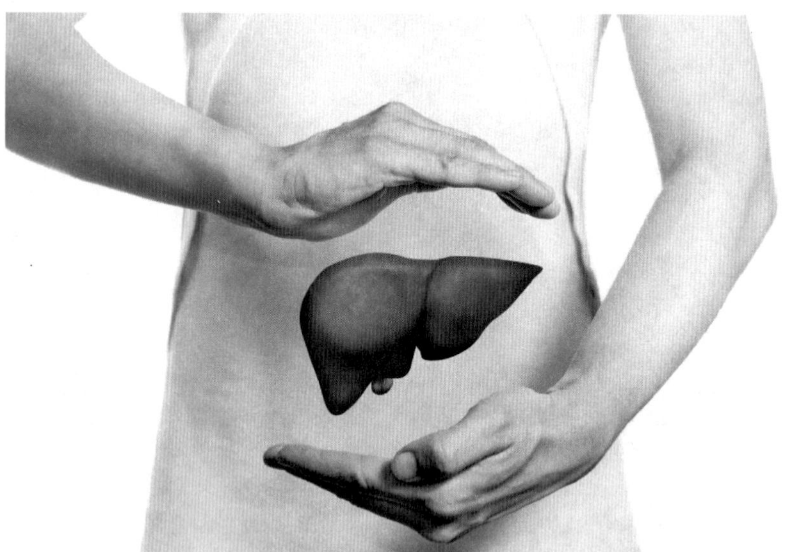

FATTY LIVER DISEASE

Besides elevation of cholesterol and triglycerides – and their adverse effects on the cardiovascular system – there are other consequences of inadequate thyroid stimulation of liver function. Specifically, in the absence of sufficient thyroid hormone, the liver fails to metabolize fats properly. This results in a condition called nonalcoholic fatty liver disease or NAFLD. In cases where this backup of fats causes an inflammatory response in the liver, it can progress to nonalcoholic steatohepatitis (NASH). About 10% of patients with NASH progress to cirrhosis and end-stage liver disease. And that's not a very happy ending, I'm afraid.

According to MayoClinic.org:[90]

> *"NAFLD is increasingly common around the world, especially in Western nations. In the United States, it's the most common form of chronic liver disease, affecting about one-quarter of the population."*

And like so many other conditions that are due to hypofunction of metabolism – but never identified as such due to "normal" TSH levels – the cause remains a mystery to Ivory Tower academicians in charge of teaching medical students. "Experts don't know exactly why some people accumulate fat in the liver while others do not," states the MayoClinic.org writer. However, the site does identify some risk factors that sound very familiar to those of us who have learned to diagnose and treat hypothyroidism by clinical assessment. Those risk factors are the following: high cholesterol, high triglycerides, metabolic syndrome, obesity, polycystic ovarian syndrome, sleep apnea, type 2 diabetes, underactive thyroid, underactive pituitary, and old age.

It's no coincidence that the risk factors for fatty liver are nearly the same as the symptoms of hypothyroidism. Sinha, Singh, and Yen[91] discussed that in their 2018 paper: "potential application of thyroid hormones and/or thyroid hormone analogues for the treatment of hypercholesterolaemia and non-alcoholic fatty liver disease (NAFLD)." In conclusion, they state:

> *"Advances in our understanding of the cellular and molecular mechanisms of fatty acid and cholesterol synthesis and metabolism have led to a better appreciation for the role of thyroid hormones and THRs in maintaining normal hepatic lipid homeostasis…the new advances in our knowledge in these areas that are presented in this Review provide stronger*

> *rationales and tools for using thyroid hormone or thyromimetic drugs to treat hepatic metabolic disorders."*

How about that! I haven't had many patients who know that they have fatty liver, and I certainly didn't screen for it, so I can't offer any personal experience in this area. But my strong suspicion is that if one were to evaluate my well-replaced patients for fatty liver, one would find very few cases, much fewer than 25%. Hopefully, someone will do such a study someday.

SLUGGISH CLEARANCE OF DRUGS, ESTROGEN, PCOS

Another critical function of the liver is metabolizing, conjugating, burning, and detoxifying various substances in the bloodstream. This applies to both endogenously produced substances like our hormones and exogenous substances like drugs, alcohol, and toxins. Hypothyroid patients are often very sensitive to prescription drugs. They tend to get side effects easily and frequently, and they often have learned that they need a far smaller dose of whatever drug they might be given to get the desired result. In addition, hypothyroid patients are commonly very sensitive to alcohol and caffeine. When hypothyroid, many of my patients had already voluntarily discontinued alcohol and caffeine because they had become overly sensitive to their effects due to their declining thyroid function.

Another common example of this sensitivity is in the metabolism and clearance of estrogen. We know that the ovaries of women of reproductive age produce estrogen continuously. The production amount varies throughout the menstrual cycle, but production occurs daily, nonetheless. Well, if estrogen is being pumped into the bloodstream daily, where does it go? Why does the level not continue to rise higher and higher?

The answer, of course, is that the estrogen is constantly being conjugated and thus removed by the liver. It's converted to estrogenically inactive metabolites, which are then excreted in the urine or the stool via the biliary tract. In their 2005 paper, Tsuchiya, Nakajima, and Yokoi[92] explain:

> *"The first step in this metabolism of estrogens is the hydroxylation catalyzed by cytochrome P450 (CYP) enzymes. Since most CYP isoforms are abundantly expressed in liver, the metabolism of estrogens mainly occurs in the liver."*

When thyroid isn't adequate, this liver function is reduced. As a result, estrogen is broken down more slowly, and we see higher levels of estrogen in the blood.

Then, exactly as we'd expect, the parts of the body that are stimulated by estrogen, like the uterine lining, become *overstimulated.* Periods get heavier and heavier because the endometrium grows thicker with every cycle because it's overstimulated with estrogen that isn't being deactivated and cleared by the liver. This can, of course, increase the risk of endometrial cancer, which may explain why three well-known risk factors associated with increased risk of endometrial cancer are obesity, diabetes, and hypertension. They don't *cause* cancer per se; I believe they're associated with endometrial cancer because hypothyroidism also causes all three of those conditions. I believe underlying hypothyroidism causes all of these conditions, which is why they are frequently seen together.

Further, the regular ovulatory cycling system is eventually shut off when the estrogen level becomes too high. Ovulation will not be triggered unless there is a sufficient mid-cycle dip in estrogen level. This doesn't happen if estrogen isn't being cleared adequately from the bloodstream by the liver. This persistence of a high estrogen level in the bloodstream is also why pregnancy and birth control pills turn off ovulation. When the estrogen level gets this high due to hypothyroidism, we then have oligomenorrhea (infrequent periods) and even full anovulation (no periods at all).

If infrequent or absent periods sound familiar, they should. That's what we currently call "polycystic ovarian syndrome," or PCOS. To be precise, PCOS refers to a condition in women of childbearing age where ovulation is infrequent or absent. Frequently, there's also evidence of excess androgen production, such as excess hair (hirsutism) and acne. In addition, the ovaries are often covered with small follicle cysts, ovulations that never made it to fruition. Thus, the name "polycystic ovarian syndrome." PCOS is a common condition in women between 18 and 44 and is a preventable cause of infertility. Interestingly, PCOS is not new. It was first described in Italy in 1721.

You might ask, why is there excess androgen production in these women? The answer can be found in the organic chemistry I studied in medical school. Whenever there is a significant excess accumulation of estrogen, some excess estrogen essentially "spills over" and proceeds down the biochemical enzymatic pathway to form androgens. The structure of estrogen and androgens are quite similar, so it does not take much excess estrogen for some of that to be converted into testosterone and other androgens.

Doctors understood that anovulation should be treated with thyroid hormone in the first half of the 20th century. By the time I was trained in the 1970s, that simple fix was no longer taught. Instead, Stein-Leventhal Syndrome – what we called PCOS back then – was a mysterious condition of the ovaries with an unknown cause. Women who weren't trying to conceive were "treated" with birth control pills. Those who wanted a baby were treated with a "wedge resection," where part of the ovary was surgically "wedged out."

Fortunately, there is a glimmer of hope that modern medicine may eventually be able to understand this condition. The Wikipedia listing for PCOS[93] starts by saying, "PCOS is a heterogeneous disorder of uncertain cause." But it goes on to say:

> *"PCOS has some aspects of a metabolic disorder, since its symptoms are partly reversible. Even though considered as a gynecological problem, PCOS consists of 28 clinical symptoms…recent insights show a multisystem disorder, with the primary problem lying in hormonal regulation in the hypothalamus, with the involvement of many organs."*

And as one might predict, those 28 symptoms again sound very similar to a list of symptoms of hypothyroidism. At this point, are you surprised?

CHAPTER 11: EFFECTS ON REPRODUCTIVE HEALTH

"Women complain about premenstrual syndrome, but I think of it as the only time of the month that I can be myself."
~ Roseanne Barr

Hormones in women are highly interconnected, and low levels of thyroid hormone can dramatically affect fertility, pregnancy, libido, and menstrual health. Let's look at some of these crucial connections.

INFERTILITY AND HYPERPROLACTINEMIA

Over years of treating women with hypothyroidism, I've been able to help dozens of young women get pregnant by optimizing their thyroid treatment, which normalized their irregular periods. That's immensely gratifying for the patients – and also for me! Better yet, the patient gets a substantial financial bonus! Monthly thyroid medication costs much less than a cycle or two of *in vitro* fertilization!

Thyroid hormone was one of the first infertility treatments used by doctors starting in the mid-twentieth century. Sadly, the full text of that literature isn't easy to find. Still, a search of "use of thyroid for infertility" at Pubmed.gov[94] lists a collection of articles with titles including: "Thyroid extract versus thyroxine: critical evaluation with particular reference to functional infertility" (1950); "Evaluation of thyroid in the treatment of sterility" (1952); "Some aspects of thyroid function in relation to infertility" (1947); "Effect of thyroid therapy on menstrual disorders and sterility" (1954); and "Male infertility treated with desiccated thyroid: case report" (1957).

A 2006 review article by Trokoudes, Skordis, and Picolos[95] reports that:

> *"Thyroid dysfunction…interferes with human reproductive physiology, reduces the likelihood of pregnancy and adversely affects pregnancy outcome…Subclinical hypothyroidism may be associated with ovulatory dysfunction…Awareness of the thyroid status in the infertile couple is crucial because of its significant frequent and often reversible or preventable effect on infertility."*

An Iranian study from 1975[96] describes a trial of thyroid replacement in 24 infertility patients who had problems with post-ovulatory progesterone production, known as a luteal phase deficiency. Half of the patients were treated with thyroid, and the other half were given a placebo. The study reported that

> *"The incidence of pregnancy in the group taking thyroid hormone was much higher, which suggests that a course of thyroid hormone should be administered before a more aggressive therapy with chorionic gonadotropins or Clomid is given."*

In 1991, a Japanese study[97] reported a case of a 37-year-old woman with long-standing amenorrhea, galactorrhea (lactation in the absence of recent pregnancy), and pituitary enlargement. The woman received thyroid treatment, resolved her symptoms, and normalized her prolactin level and pituitary size. Like the Iranian authors, the researchers recommended that "thyroid hormone replacement should be a first-choice therapy preceding the pituitary surgery or bromocriptine therapy." In 1992, Israeli researchers[98] reported on two similar cases, one of whom was even spared from planned pituitary surgery because her pituitary returned to normal size with thyroid replacement. (My guess is that she was pleased about that!)

The Japanese team of Abe and Momotani[99] summarized it best in their 1997 review article (in Japanese) when they wrote the following:

> *"Thyroid disorders have been implicated in a broad spectrum of reproductive disorders ranging from abnormal sexual development to menstrual irregularities and infertility…Long-standing, untreated hypothyroidism is associated with galactorrhea. These abnormalities are reversible with adequate thyroid supplementation…thus, during the investigation of hirsutism, menstrual irregularity, infertility, galactorrhea, and gynecomastia, the possibility of thyroid dysfunction must always be considered."*

The only question I have is this: Where are the American researchers? Why do we have to go all around the world to find these articles? I suspect American physicians were increasingly pressured to manage thyroid by lab tests, so trials would not be considered unless an abnormal TSH permitted them even to diagnose hypothyroidism and then prescribe thyroid to these women. So, thyroid treatment was never even considered if a patient with infertility had a normal TSH. As a result, the practice of empirically giving thyroid for problems with infertility fell out of fashion due to the rise of the almighty TSH. This is yet another example of the lost art of medicine due to this misguided, foolish, yet widespread belief that the TSH measures thyroid function.

EFFECTS ON PREGNANCY

We have already discussed the association of hypothyroidism with infertility due to ovulation abnormalities. Often the abnormalities in ovulation are resolved by proper thyroid replacement, and pregnancy is achieved. The problem is that once pregnancy is confirmed, the mother and her child aren't free of the adverse effects of maternal hypothyroidism. Sadly, hypothyroidism can complicate pregnancy in many ways.

Many authors over many years have noted associations of overt hypothyroidism as well as "sub-clinical hypothyroidism" (elevated TSH with normal T3 and T4) and "thyroid autoimmunity" (presence of thyroid peroxidase antibodies in the serum) with increased rates of abnormalities. These include low birth weight and fetal distress,[100] miscarriage, preterm delivery, hypertension in pregnancy,[101] neurologic impairment and reduced IQ in the infant,[102] intrauterine growth retardation,[103] and even breech presentation.[104]

According to Debanjali Sarkar's literature review of 2012,[105]

> *"Autoimmune thyroid disease is present in around 4% of young females, and up to 15% are at risk because they are thyroid antibody-positive. There is a strong relationship between thyroid immunity on one hand and infertility, miscarriage, and thyroid disturbances in pregnancy and postpartum, on the other hand. Even minimal hypothyroidism can increase rates of miscarriage and fetal death and may also have adverse effects on later cognitive development of the offspring."*

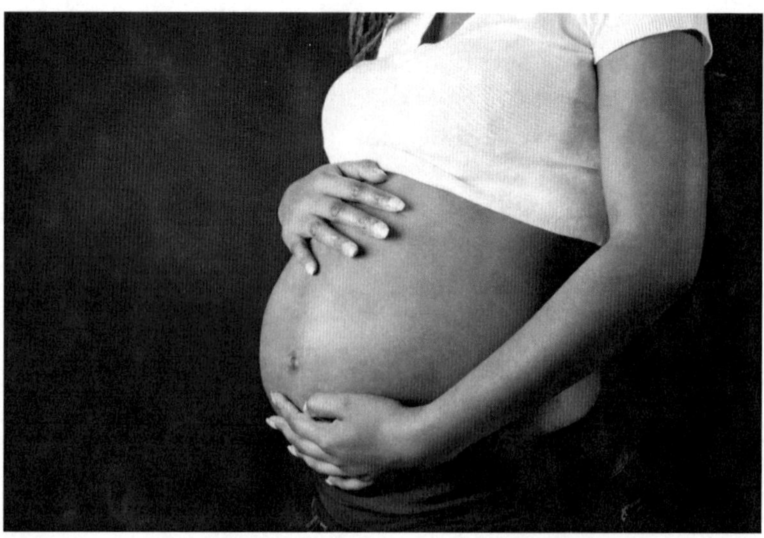

In contrast to the apparent consensus among researchers that thyroid dysfunction is associated with multiple pregnancy complications, there seems to be great disagreement among those same researchers about the best management of these pregnant patients to reduce the chance of adverse outcomes. The TABLET RCT[106] (The **T**hyroid **A**nti**B**odies and **LE**vo**T**hyroxine **R**andomized **C**ontrolled **T**rial) was a multicentered randomized, double-blind placebo-controlled trial performed in the UK between 2011 and 2016. The study aimed to determine whether thyroid replacement reduced complications in pregnant women with normal TSH but elevated thyroid peroxidase antibodies. The study randomized subjects to receive either 50 mcg of levothyroxine daily or a placebo and pregnancy outcomes were measured. Researchers studied 540 pregnancies, concluding that "levothyroxine therapy in a dose of 50 mcg per day does not improve the live birth rate in euthyroid women with thyroid peroxidase antibodies." This outcome is certainly not surprising since they used a one-size-fits-all approach with a tiny dose of thyroid, a dose that is unlikely to adequately fulfill most patients' thyroid requirements.

Another study from 2016 by Kattah and Garovic[107] looked at the relationship between subclinical hypothyroidism and gestational hypertension. They concluded that "there is no strong evidence to support treating patients with subclinical hypothyroidism and hypertension solely to improve blood pressure control." In contrast, during the same year, Ramtahal and Dhanoo[108] published a case report of a 25-year-old woman having her first pregnancy. She had hypertension, an elevated TSH, a normal T4, and was positive for thyroid peroxidase antibodies. She was diagnosed with subclinical hypothyroidism. They found that "the patient was successfully treated with levothyroxine which normalized the blood pressure without the need for antihypertensive treatment."

Finally, two extensive literature reviews, one in 2013 by Velkeniers, Meerhaeghe, et al.[109] and the other in 2019 by Rao, Zeng, Zhou, et al.,[110] concluded from their reviews that "LT4 supplementation should be recommended to improve clinical pregnancy outcome in women with subclinical hypothyroidism." Specifically, they found that giving thyroid hormone to women with subclinical hypothyroidism resulted in significantly higher live birth rates and a significant decrease in both pregnancy loss and preterm birth rates.

Given all the confusion within the literature, what's a doctor to do when a hypothyroid woman gets pregnant? Well, my answer is to ideally have their dose optimized before conception and then keep it that way throughout the pregnancy to optimize fetal brain development and minimize pregnancy complications. But because pregnancy is such a high-intensity, risky situation in a world full of underemployed lawyers, and because I have avoided hospitals for many years, I was able to refer my patients to a friendly endocrinologist who managed my patients' thyroid needs during their pregnancies. This particular endocrinologist had become relatively open-minded about thyroid doses, and he generally allowed my pregnant patients to continue on their pre-referral doses. Even if these patients had suppressed TSH levels, he allowed them to continue as long as they looked and felt well on those doses. Since he regularly saw hospitalized patients, other doctors in the hospital – including the obstetricians – knew him, trusted him, and accepted his thyroid management without question. With his gracious assistance, my patients had good outcomes and relatively uncomplicated pregnancies.

Unfortunately, about 8 years ago, there was an exception. A patient in her 30s had difficulty conceiving, but with proper thyroid replacement, she was able to conceive and was carrying twins. During the first trimester, she moved from the DC area to North Carolina and found an obstetrician there. She was looking and doing well and was perfectly stable on her dose when she left and had no signs or symptoms of overdose. But sadly, her obstetric team in North Carolina found it entirely unacceptable that her TSH was suppressed on the thyroid dose that had helped her conceive, and they insisted that she reduce the dose in half. Not knowing there were other options, she did as they insisted. Shortly after that, she miscarried the twins at 14 weeks gestation.

Several months later, I heard this sad news when she returned to see me again to get her dose back on track. We got her back on a good thyroid dose, and she happily conceived again quite quickly.

But this time, she found a new obstetrician in North Carolina who agreed to be more open-minded about her thyroid dose and allowed her to stay on her therapeutic dose. Nine months later, she had an uncomplicated vaginal delivery of a healthy, beautiful, blue-eyed, blond-haired baby boy. She brought him to see me for a follow-up visit 18 months later. I'll never forget meeting this young man. Before his mom's visit, he had been playing with Lego pieces in the reception area. When he walked back into my office with his mom, he approached me behind my desk without hesitation and carefully placed a Lego propeller onto my desk. He then looked and me and said the word "FLY"! I was almost speechless! This 18-month-old young man was clearly very bright, and I can't help but think it may have something to do with the thyroid dose stimulating his brain development for those nine months! It was a wonderful day for me and a terrific outcome for this patient and her smart son (who will probably grow up to be a rocket scientist or find the cure for cancer someday! Better yet, perhaps he will invent a blood test that directly measures metabolic rate!)

Interestingly, delivery isn't the end of pregnancy-related issues that can occur with thyroid function. It turns out that pregnancy itself is often a cause of thyroid dysfunction, such as the condition known as postpartum thyroiditis. According to Argatska and Nonchev's 2014 paper:[111]

> *"Postpartum thyroiditis is a syndrome of transient or permanent thyroid dysfunction occurring in the first year after delivery or abortion. It is the most common thyroid disease in the postpartum period, with incidence between 5 and 9%. In essence, it is an autoimmune inflammation of the thyroid, caused by changes in humoral and cell-mediated immune response."*

One might expect that a significant number of women who develop post-partum thyroiditis might develop postpartum depression since depression is a prominent symptom of hypothyroidism. In reviewing the literature, I found only scant data linking the two. And since I haven't done obstetrics in over three decades, I have not seen or managed a patient with postpartum depression in a very long time. When I did take care of obstetric patients who developed postpartum depression, I knew almost nothing about thyroid function other than to diagnose and manage it by lab tests, as we all had been taught.

However, knowing what I know now, if I were ever in the position of taking care of a patient with postpartum depression, which can be a very dangerous condition, I would undoubtedly evaluate that patient closely for other clinical symptoms or signs of hypothyroidism. I would be highly likely to give that patient a trial of thyroid replacement since that condition is otherwise quite hard to control and can threaten the lives of both the patient and her baby.

The other common consequence of post-partum thyroiditis is permanent hypothyroidism. Many of my hypothyroid patients reported being perfectly well until they delivered a child. Then, they suddenly started gaining weight, became extremely tired, lost their hair, and developed sleep problems. These symptoms were more extreme than the health challenges that many women face when raising a newborn. I don't exactly understand how pregnancy changes in a woman's immune system can alter thyroid function, but it seems to happen frequently. In addition, what is even stranger, I have seen maybe a dozen women give a history of sudden onset of symptoms of hypothyroidism in response to having had a hysterectomy with or without removal of the ovaries and without any surgical complications causing massive blood loss that could have caused any pituitary damage. (We touched on this phenomenon earlier in the discussion on estrogen.) I have found no literature to support this observation, but I have seen this association quite a few times and would feel remiss by not mentioning it. If you have also seen this association, please contact me!

BREAST SORENESS

Breast pain is a common condition, particularly premenstrually. Breast soreness is yet another consequence of allowing the estrogen level in the blood to get too high. My traditional gynecology training taught me that uncomfortable breast soreness should be treated with diuretics, salt restriction, antidepressants, analgesics, or abstaining from caffeine. I now know that breast soreness usually resolves with adequate thyroid replacement. It's the same mechanism as thyroid replacement reducing the volume and intensity of heavy periods. It turns out that if you wake up the liver with thyroid, estrogen is metabolized and cleared out of the bloodstream faster. The symptoms of overstimulation in estrogen-dependent tissues like the breasts and the endometrium melt away. There is no need for diuretics, salt restriction, analgesics, etc. when a woman suffers from breast pain.

SEXUAL DESIRE

Another effect of hypothyroidism on a woman's reproductive function that I would like to discuss is the effect on sex drive. Sex drive is seldom spared by hypothyroidism. I've had many patients claim that their libido is "less than zero" – a *negative* value! I always try to reassure them that having a desire to have sex when one hasn't had a thoroughly restful night of sleep in years would seem a bit out of place. And let's not discount that 30 pounds of weight gain can make many women reluctant to be seen naked! Sadly, low libido is also one of the most challenging symptoms to reverse with thyroid replacement. I didn't keep detailed statistics, but I estimate that my success rate for fixing low libido with thyroid replacement – and adding estrogen replacement if deficient – was only about 50%. Of course, that is better than no chance of improvement, but the resolution of low libido is never something that should be guaranteed. Perhaps that has to do with the fact that libido is a very elusive and multifactorial quality in women, affected by many things besides hormones.

At the other end of the spectrum, what is most interesting is that hypersexuality can be a symptom – albeit rare – of thyroid overdose. I have seen a handful of women who have complained of hypersexuality due to being on too much thyroid. (Perhaps more were affected but didn't complain?) The first patient who reported such an effect was a 72-year-old, widowed, retired schoolteacher. She had no partner at that time, so this was a problem for her, but it was resolved quickly with a reduction of her dose. Interestingly, she is now happily remarried and thoroughly enjoying her married life with her new husband.

PMS (PREMENSTRUAL SYNDROME) / PMDD (PREMENSTRUAL DYSPHORIC DISORDER)

Finally, let's talk about periods. Menstruation, the "curse," "Aunt Flo" – whatever you call it – it's an unavoidable part of life for most women, from adolescence until menopause. Hypothyroidism significantly impacts menstrual cycles, premenstrual symptoms, and other menstrual problems.

Wikipedia[112] has a decent definition of premenstrual syndrome:

> *"Premenstrual Syndrome (PMS) refers to emotional and physical symptoms that regularly occur in the one to two weeks before the start of each menstrual period. Symptoms resolve around the start of bleeding. Different women experience different symptoms. The common emotional symptoms include irritability and mood changes while the common physical symptoms include acne, tender breasts, bloating, and feeling tired; these are also seen in women without PMS. Often symptoms are present for around six days. An individual's pattern of symptoms may change over time. Symptoms do not occur during pregnancy or following menopause."*

And, as we expect, they add the following: "The cause of PMS is unknown," adding that this condition affects "20 to 30% of menstruating women."

During my gynecologic post-graduate training, I was taught that PMS – affectionately referred to by some as "Poor Me Syndrome" – was a mysterious condition of unknown etiology in many menstruating women. These patients suffered each month with extreme symptoms of emotional lability, irritability, water retention, weight gain, hunger, depression, breast pain, etc., usually occurring during the two weeks before their periods. The symptoms classically resolved with the onset of the woman's period. The most severe form of this is called Premenstrual

Dysphoric Disorder, or PMDD, which is so severe that it qualifies as its own distinct psychiatric condition. In 2013, PMDD was classified in the Diagnostic and Statistical Manual of Mental Disorders. Its official code in that manual is DSM-5 625.4 (N94.3).

Even the World Health Organization jumped into the fray. As of June 2019, PMDD has been added to the eleventh revision of the International Statistical Classification of Diseases and Related Health Problems classification system, the ICD-11 coding system.[113] These are the codes that insurance companies require if one wants to get them to pay for one's healthcare. The ICD-11 Code for PMDD is GA34.41.

PMDD even has its own association, "The International Association for Premenstrual Disorders (IAPMD)."[114] The organization describes itself as "the leading voluntary health organization which aspires to create a world where people with Premenstrual Dysphoric Disorder (PMDD) and Premenstrual exacerbation (PME) can survive and thrive. Our mission is to inspire hope and end suffering in those affected by Premenstrual Disorders." As one might expect, IAPMD is thrilled with this classification achievement since it "validate[s] PMDD as a legitimate medical diagnosis worldwide and acknowledge[es] our growing scientific and medical understanding of this little known but debilitating condition."

The only problem is that we continue to have little actual scientific and medical understanding of PMDD. For example, they state the following:

> *"Twenty years of experimental research has revealed that…hormone levels and patterns appear normal in those with PMDD…Menopause is the only 'cure' for PMDD…and mounting evidence indicates that PMDD is caused by a biological brain difference and can be treated using biological interventions."*

Great! "A biological brain difference!" That really clarifies things, doesn't it?!

Miles E Drake, Jr, MD, writes at Theravive[115] that "the new diagnosis has not been without controversy, as feminist writers have argued that this amounts to the medicalization of some women's normal bodily phenomena.[116] The association of menstrual periods with mood disturbance, emotional changes, and neurovegetative symptoms has been recognized since the time of Hippocrates, when menstrual bleeding was thought to "purge melancholic and choleric humors."[117]

As for an explanation of the pathophysiology of this condition, Dr. Drake continues:

> *"The organic cause of PMDD is now generally accepted but not definitely established, and an association between hormonal fluctuations of the menstrual cycle and neurotransmitter disturbances involved in depression is suspected."*

I don't know about you, but that description doesn't exactly explain what is going on other than saying, "Her fluctuating hormones are making her crazy!" Any husband or partner could have told us that! Yet, the IAPMD states that hormone levels are normal. Hmm. Not very illuminating, for sure. Dr. Drake goes on to discuss treatment as follows: "Treatment focuses on regularization of menses, amelioration of symptoms and repair of disrupted social relationships." So "there's something wrong with her hormones" and "you should treat her individual symptoms and offer couples counseling."

How about treating the underlying hormonal disturbance with a hormonal treatment?!

Gynecologists have used many therapies over the years to try to treat PMS. They range from birth control pills to diuretics, vitamins, antidepressants and mood stabilizers, progesterone creams, lotions, and potions. I even had one patient, a psychologist, who used progesterone-in-oil rectal suppositories for PMS, and she swore that it helped. Sarafem is a product specifically designed to treat PMS, and it's nothing more than Prozac (Fluoxetine) packaged in a girly-looking pink and lavender capsule. None of these has been a reliable treatment for everyone with

PMS. All of these products work to some extent to control the various symptoms, but none directly addresses the root of the problem.

Here's a clue. According to Drugs.com,[118] the symptoms caused by excess progesterone are drowsiness, dizziness, breast pain, mood changes, headache, constipation, diarrhea, bloating, swelling, and a few others. In addition, according to Dovemed.com,[119] the symptoms of excess estrogen are breast tenderness, fluid retention, dramatic changes in mood and temperament, drowsiness, headache, and a few others.

Could it be that PMS is related to elevated levels of estrogen and progesterone during the luteal phase – the two weeks before a period – in a menstruating woman?

And, as we discussed earlier, what happens to the levels of those two hormones if a woman cannot metabolize, and thus clear out, her own hormones? Bingo! Even MORE excess!

Indeed, PMS seems to be due to an exaggeration of the normal elevations of estrogen and progesterone that occurs during the luteal phase of a woman's period. And that explains why the symptoms of PMS almost always resolve with the onset of the woman's period because the start signifies that the hormone levels have dropped enough for that period to occur.

Bear with me here. Let's say that the symptoms of PMS are due to excess accumulation of estrogen and progesterone during the two weeks prior to a woman's period, due to sluggish metabolism of those hormones by the liver, and those symptoms go away when the hormone levels drop. Isn't it reasonable to think that adding thyroid hormone, which speeds up the clearance of those hormones, could *also* relieve PMS symptoms? Couldn't we use thyroid hormone to "flatten the curve" of those hormones, as one might say in the age of Covid?

Absolutely! And, of course, that is precisely what happens! In my experience, after trying just about every possible medicine that has ever been suggested for treating PMS, thyroid replacement seems to work the best and most reliably to relieve those symptoms. So, thyroid is my choice to treat symptoms of PMS and PMDD. And my patients – and their loved ones – were always very grateful for this simple cure!

I'm not the first to make this discovery. Broda Barnes alluded to these benefits on page 125 of his book.[120] He reported that thyroid replacement relieves the following symptoms: "undue fatigue…requiring more than the usual amount of sleep and yet awakening tired…being nervous, irritable, easily upset by insignificant incidents." (That sounds a lot like PMS to me!)

Yet, if you do a medical literature search, you will surprisingly not find many others who have written about this phenomenon. A 1990 article published in the *Journal of Clinical Endocrinology and Metabolism*[121] referenced a 1986 study that reported the following:

> *"It was reported that a high percentage of women with premenstrual syndrome (PMS) were found to have thyroid hypofunction (TH), mostly subclinical hypothyroidism, as defined by an augmented response of TSH to TRH, and that all affected women had complete relief of PMS symptoms with L-T4 therapy."*

I was unable to locate that original source article. Nonetheless, based on my own experience, I would encourage anyone with PMS or PMDD to be given a trial of thyroid replacement as a first-line treatment since it usually works like a charm, and there's very little to lose by doing a trial.

I can't help but think back to a patient, a lovely and intelligent 28-year-old cybersecurity specialist. I had an initial visit with her not long before I retired. She had suffered from incapacitating PMS her entire reproductive life. She had seen many specialists, received many worrisome and incorrect diagnoses, and spent the equivalent of a monthly mortgage payment on various drugs and supplements to treat her symptoms. I had her begin a thyroid trial.

Before my retirement, I saw her for a follow-up visit, and she told me she was enjoying a significant improvement in her PMS symptoms! That's gratifying, but what remains frustrating is that I was the *first* doctor even to offer her a trial of thyroid hormone. I look forward to a time when more doctors look to thyroid replacement as a ready solution for various reproductive challenges that so many women needlessly suffer.

CHAPTER 12: NEUROLOGIC SYMPTOMS AND MENTAL HEALTH

"For the past ten days, I've had a migraine that follows me like a shadow. One hundred and forty-two hours of incessant pain, an eight on the ten-point scale. I have a CT scan, an MRI, I go to the neurologist—the readings are all inconclusive. I'm told it's a migraine with an unknown cause. 'Have you tried yoga?' they say."
~ Karla Cornejo Villavicencio

Hypothyroidism is very interrelated with the neurologic system as well as mental health. Let's look at some common neurologic conditions and symptoms that can benefit from thyroid hormone.

MIGRAINE

Migraine or migraine headaches are likely caused by vasomotor spasms in the brain and in the vascular tissues covering the brain (the meninges). These are sometimes referred to as vasomotor headaches. One well-known trigger for migraine in women is a sudden drop in estrogen levels, such as the drop that occurs right before the start of a menstrual period. As discussed earlier in Chapter 3, a sudden drop in estrogen level will precipitate vasospasms in the blood vessels. And when the vessels in the brain and meninges have spasms, throbbing and intense pain can occur. When a woman experiences a migraine before her period, it's appropriately called "menstrual migraine," The condition even has its unique diagnostic code. It's also fairly common for menstrual migraines to resolve after menopause when a woman's natural monthly hormonal fluctuations subside.

It sounds a bit complicated, but the bottom line is this: relatively sudden but natural drops in the estrogen level that occur just before a woman's period can trigger vasospasms, and those vasospasms can manifest as migraine. In addition, the larger the fluctuation in the hormone levels, the more likely a migraine will occur.

Many hypothyroid women have migraines, particularly those with icy hands. The old saying "cold hands, warm heart" would be more accurate if it were changed to "cold hands, achy head." I believe part of the reason for this is that the hypothyroid body, which has, by definition, a slow metabolism, is simply not producing enough heat to heat the entire body. To conserve heat, the blood vessels near the body's surface constrict. This is most noticeable in the extremities and the brain.

Interestingly, a Finnish study described this association between coldness and migraines in an article published in 2014.[122] The authors reported a statistically significant reduction in the surface temperature of five peripheral sites, including the nose and hands, among migraine patients compared to non-migraineur controls. They hypothesized that the "peripheral coldness [was] possibly due to abnormal autonomic vascular control."

Indeed. Dr. Alexander Mauskop, a prominent neurologist/headache specialist in New York City and the author of the "New York Headache Blog,"[123] confirms this association between migraine headaches and "coldness of hands and feet or just feeling colder in general than other people in the same environment." But sadly, he doesn't go one step more to make the association between low thyroid function and coldness.

There's another reason why migraines may be more problematic in hypothyroid women. The sudden drop in estrogen level appears to be intensified in many hypothyroid patients. As we discussed earlier, this is likely due to exaggerated peaks and valleys in the hormone levels of these women due to slowed estrogen clearance by the sluggish hypothyroid liver.

The good news is that this is easy to fix with thyroid treatment and sometimes adding some estrogen around the onset of the periods in menstruating women.

I believe that thyroid replacement works for migraine the same way it warms up cold hands and feet and makes skin and hair healthier. Adding thyroid hormone increases the metabolic rate, and this increases heat production. Since the body is now warmer, it no longer needs to conserve heat so intensely. Therefore, the peripheral blood vessels can open up and let warm blood flow freely to the hands, feet, skin, scalp, hair follicles, and brain. Warm, free-flowing blood in the brain helps prevent vasospasms, reducing the cause of the migraine.

In addition, adding thyroid to a menstruating woman will increase the clearance of the reproductive hormones that are cycling each month, so the peaks will not be so high, and the drop in the estrogen level before the period will not be so extreme. It's pretty simple, and it's a shame that we aren't taught how to do this during our medical training. I would estimate that about 90% of my patients with migraine had complete resolution when they reached a dose of thyroid that caused their hands and feet to warm up.

In some cases, estrogen can come to the rescue if thyroid treatment isn't enough. My approach was to give some estrogen to those women for a few days before the onset of the period and then for the first several days to prevent the estrogen level from dropping too low. For years, menopause practitioners like myself have been preventing menstrual migraines by supplementing estrogen just during periods, usually using estrogen patches. We simply have a patient put on a 0.1 mg estrogen patch a day or two *before* she thinks a menstrual migraine will start and then discontinues the patch four to seven days later, as the estrogen level naturally begins to climb. That usually prevents menstrual migraine because the trough of the natural estrogen curve is filled in a bit by the estrogen from the patch.

Consequently, the amplitude of the cyclic fall in the estrogen level is smaller and thus less intense. The blood vessels are less disturbed and spasm less, thereby preventing migraine. Better living through creative hormonal physiology!

The ability to cure chronic migraine headaches is often one of the easiest and most rewarding results of replacing thyroid properly. Chronic migraines are tremendously debilitating, and current standard treatments include some medicines with potential risks and procedures like Botox injections that, in too many cases, offer limited control of the problem or are cost-prohibitive for many migraineurs. To completely cure a patient's tendency to have migraine headaches is a gift, and I am very grateful to have been able to do this for my migraine patients. It can be life-changing!

MOOD, COGNITION, AND CRAVINGS

Depression, anxiety, and "foggy brain" are widespread symptoms in hypothyroid patients. As mentioned earlier, the brain cells are covered with thyroid and estrogen receptors. It appears that optimal brain function depends on good thyroid – and, again, estrogen – function. Based on the evaluation of cognitive and mood symptoms reported by hypothyroid patients, that certainly seems to be the case. Further, it's well established that proper fetal and childhood brain development is dependent on the presence of adequate thyroid function.

Cretinism is the name of the condition where the developing fetus either lacks a thyroid gland, the thyroid gland isn't receiving proper stimulation from the hypothalamus, or severe maternal iodine deficiency is present. This condition is more common in mountainous areas like the Himalayas and inland China, and also Africa, where iodine is deficient in the soil and the food.[124] The hallmark finding in cretinism is profound mental retardation and delayed cognitive development. IQs tend to be in the 60 range. In fact, "iodine deficiency is the most common preventable cause of brain damage in the world."[125] These individuals usually die prematurely due to complications of various developmental abnormalities. Adequate thyroid function is crucial to the development of the human brain and extremely important to human development in general.

Thus, it's no surprise that cognition is also frequently compromised in adults with clinical hypothyroidism. My patients often described their inability to concentrate, inability to focus, and poor memory and recall as "brain fog" or "foggy brain." (Estrogen is also a player here, but my impression is that thyroid deficiency is the more important of the two. Ideally, both should be adequately replaced.)

Sometimes the brain fog is so bad that patients retire early or have even gone out on disability because they can't focus enough to work. Not uncommonly, by the time patients come to see me, they are already on various medications for diagnoses like ADD, depression, anxiety, etc. Interestingly, Wellbutrin is often the antidepressant used to treat depression in hypothyroid patients, probably because of its stimulant effect. If you press these patients about their depression, their primary complaint is not sadness. Instead, it's more often exhaustion and lack of energy to do anything that might be enjoyable. They are just too tired to be happy. The concept of going out to do something fun is simply overwhelming. Sometimes this lack of motivation can be quite disabling. Some patients eventually become withdrawn, hopeless, and occasionally even suicidal, particularly after seeing dozens of doctors who have all assured them, based solely on lab tests, that their thyroid is just fine and that they are just depressed. I would also be hopeless if all I could see in my future were a desire to sleep, an inability to do such, and no energy to do anything.

Severely hypothyroid patients can also have paralyzing anxiety. I have had a few patients who could not leave their homes for years due to anxiety caused by hypothyroidism. Anxiety is usually not nearly that profound in hypothyroid patients, but it can often be problematic. Most of my patients with significant anxiety had already sought a remedy for that symptom. They were usually on an SSRI drug or other anxiolytic drug or mood stabilizer by the time they came to see me. Often, they were able to discontinue those medicines once we found the optimal dose of thyroid.

Interestingly I had started thyroid replacement with the daughter of an endocrinologist friend (believe it or not!). After a few weeks of treatment, the only benefit she had seen at that point was that she felt much calmer than she did before we started the trial. We hadn't even identified anxiety as one of the symptoms we hoped to fix, but this was the first benefit that showed up on treatment! I'll take it! You have to start somewhere!

In addition to antidepressants, narcolepsy drugs like Provigil and Nuvigil are used in hypothyroid patients. Similarly, "sleep apnea" is a very common diagnosis among patients who are just hypothyroid. We know that sleep is an active brain function; it isn't a passive function. Specifically, sleep isn't just the absence of wakefulness. Proper communication between our hypothalamus and brainstem is required to allow us to sleep properly. Adequate thyroid is necessary to drive that communication. In addition, our thalamus becomes active during REM sleep, and the amygdala, the part of the brain that processes emotions, is also very active during REM sleep.[126]

Indeed, poor sleep, brain fog, anxiety, and depression are all very common central nervous system symptoms in my patients. What is the common thread in these conditions? Brain sluggishness. The brain just does not seem to have enough energy to work correctly. Its engine is just not turning over, in mechanical terms. All of these functions require energy, which the thyroid supplies. This brain sluggishness has even been demonstrated in a 2018 PET scan study of hypothyroid rats. The researchers found that:

> *"[The brains of hypothyroid rats] demonstrated lower global efficiency and decreased local cliquishness of the brain network.... [particularly in] the left posterior hippocampus, the right hypothalamus, pituitary, pons and medulla...... [Their conclusion was] Our research quantitatively confirms that*

> *hypothyroidism hampers brain cognitive function by causing impairment to the brain network of glucose metabolism."*[127]

So thinking is slow, energy is low, and motivation is a no-go. When thyroid function is low, patients don't even have enough energy to sleep! Interestingly, the drugs that work best in these situations are primarily stimulants in one form or another. And, of course, since thyroid hormone is the ultimate natural stimulant, it makes sense that patients who need thyroid but aren't diagnosed as such (because their lab tests are persistently normal) often end up on various man-made drugs, many of which happen to be stimulants.

It's no surprise that hypothyroid patients often self-medicate with various stimulants such as caffeine or nicotine to help manage some of their symptoms. Both are brain stimulants and can give the user a brief energy boost. Eating carbohydrates can serve the same purpose. This phenomenon is undeniable in patients taking levothyroxine only once daily in the morning. If you bother to ask, most of them will admit that they seem to "crash" or "hit a brick wall" around 2 to 3 p.m. That's when their morning dose wears off. Patients report losing their ability to think or concentrate at that time. So, they get a coffee, a soda, a snack, or a cigarette for a mid-afternoon pick-me-up. That usually gets them through the next several hours until they finally get home from work and crash on the sofa for their evening nap. Not an ideal routine.

Patients are constantly amazed when their cravings for these substances miraculously disappear after their thyroid hormone is properly replaced. The key to this miracle is adequate dosing but, most importantly, adding a second dose at lunchtime. Assuming they took their first dose at around 6 to 7 a.m., that morning dose usually wears off after about eight hours, so the second dose taken at lunchtime kicks in just as the first dose is wearing off. Consequently, the 3 p.m. "hitting the brick wall" phenomenon melts away, and the cravings are no longer there. It's an easy fix, and an added benefit is that they consume fewer calories, which also helps with the weight control issue that is so common.

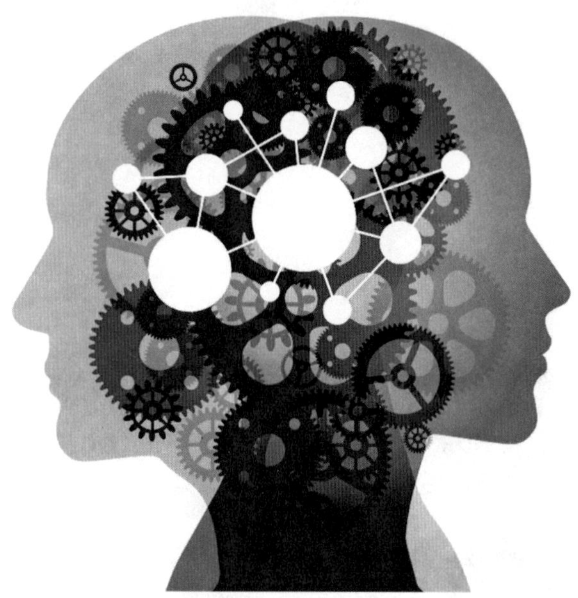

SELF-MEDICATION WITH SUBSTANCES

As I mentioned, fatigue is a common symptom in hypothyroidism, leading some women to self-medicate with stimulants, including caffeine and nicotine.

We know the dangers of smoking, and I have to say that it was gratifying to fine-tune thyroid hormone levels in smokers because after improving their overall wellness and energy levels, they often successfully quit their deadly cigarette habit. Some doctors prescribe the drug Chantix to help patients stop smoking. Chantix works by competitively binding to and stimulating the nicotine receptors in the brain. It also carries a long list of side effects and doesn't address the root cause of smoking; it simply replaces nicotine with another pharmaceutical stimulant in a less dangerous form. I would argue that directly addressing the thyroid deficiency is an infinitely better choice than either smoking or taking Chantix. (I'm sure the pharmaceutical and tobacco industries disagree!)

Given the depression and anxiety that are often symptoms of hypothyroidism, it's no surprise that alcohol is yet another substance hypothyroid patients commonly use to self-medicate. I'll defer to the experts in the fields of addiction and psychiatry to identify all the intricate nuances and reasons for this. But suffice it to say, some patients who abuse alcohol can finally control their need to drink after their thyroid is properly replaced.

I'll never forget a patient of mine from years ago. She came to me after using an endocrinologist as her primary care physician. He already had her on a once-a-day morning dose of Synthroid, and her TSH was "perfect," – but as usual, her symptoms were uncontrolled. In addition, she was a moderate to heavy drinker. Once I figured out that she needed more thyroid, she allowed me to increase her dose and have her take it morning and midday. She felt dramatically better. Then, because she felt so good, she spontaneously quit drinking successfully! Hooray!

Sometime later, however, she returned to the endocrinologist for her annual physical, and of course, he did a TSH – they can't resist – and he found it was suppressed. He convinced her that she was overdosed, even though her health had significantly improved and she had no signs or symptoms of overdose. She was so frightened by his depiction of the horrible consequences of thyroid overdose – osteoporosis, heart attack, sudden death – that she returned to her original dose. What happened next? If you guessed that she started drinking again, you would be correct. Good job, Mr. Endocrinologist! This is exactly why I firmly believe we would be much better off if the TSH test had never been invented!

SCHIZOPHRENIA

We don't often think of schizophrenia as related to hypothyroidism, but I have an interesting case to share. I had a patient, a woman around age 30, who was diagnosed with schizophrenia before I first met her. She was reasonably functional but did admit to having hallucinations fairly frequently. After seeing her for several years, I finally realized that some of her symptoms could have been due to hypothyroidism, so we started her on thyroid replacement. Somewhat amazingly, her hallucinations faded away, and the next thing I knew, she got married and had a child! What a wonderful and unexpected outcome! I remember seeing her for a routine follow-up visit, and everything was going very well for her and her family. Her dose seemed just right, and she had no hallucinations or symptoms of being underdosed or overdosed at that time.

Then, a few months later, I received a phone call from a medical student doing a rotation at a local psychiatric hospital. She told me that my patient had just been admitted to that hospital for the diagnosis of "mania." The medical student was calling because she was doing the admission history and physical exam and was unfamiliar with the drug "Armour Thyroid." Hence, she wanted to ask me about dose equivalency with levothyroxine. I told her a little bit about Armour Thyroid, but more importantly, I asked her if the patient's "manic" symptoms, by chance, included hypersexuality. As a matter of fact, they did! No doubt the student must have thought I was omniscient!

I then told her the following: "If you want to be a hero, please don't give this patient any thyroid; she will probably get better quickly!" Sure enough, three days later, I received another call, this time from the unit secretary, to inform me that my patient had gotten well and was being discharged! Hopefully, the curious and heroic medical student learned a valuable lesson about the possible effects of thyroid hormone on our emotions and behavior!

In his now out-of-print book, *Diagnosis and Management of Hypothyroidism*,[128] the late Dr. Gordon Skinner in the UK, a dear friend and colleague, described similar experiences with schizophrenia patients. He wrote:

> *"I have come across several patients deemed by more than one colleague to be schizophrenic who were cured long term by restoration of euthyroidism: a patient should never be diagnosed as schizophrenic until proper consideration has been given to hypothyroidism."*

It should be noted that when Dr. Skinner uses the word "euthyroidism," he refers to being clinically well, *not* simply having a TSH within a normal range.

I can't help but agree with Dr. Skinner's perspective. We should always consider full and proper thyroid hormone replacement for patients diagnosed with schizophrenia – not to mention migraine, mood disorders, and addictions – as a possible first step toward recovery.

CHAPTER 13: OTHER SYMPTOMS AND ISSUES

"We've been wrong about what our job is in medicine. We think our job is to ensure health and survival. But really it is larger than that. It is to enable well-being."
~ Atul Gawande, MD
from his book, "Being Mortal: Illness, Medicine and What Matters in the End"

Throughout the chapters in Part 2 of this book, I've tried to group conditions and symptoms by different physiologic systems. There are a few other symptoms and issues that didn't naturally fit in any category, but I didn't want to overlook them, so I have included them here.

COLD BODY, COLD EXTREMITIES

I've already touched upon this symptom several times in previous chapters, but feeling cold – and having cold hands and feet – is one of the most common symptoms of hypothyroidism.

That's why my patient assessments always started with observing what my patient was wearing in relation to the temperature in my office and outdoors. I remember a nearly 90-degree day in late spring when a patient came in wearing a winter coat and three pairs of pants. When I shook hands, I also paid attention to hand temperature. Was it icy? That's another classic sign.

As far as I'm concerned, these women might as well have been wearing signs on their foreheads saying, "I have no thyroid function!!!" I mentioned the thyroid-schizophrenia link earlier, and there's an intriguing point to add. Many poorly controlled schizophrenics wear multiple layers of clothing and winter coats, even in the summer. They also seem to have a strong tendency to be heavy cigarette smokers or users of other substances. For example, smoking prevalence in this population is estimated to be 80 to 90%.[129] Perhaps they are trying to tell us something about thyroid deficiency as well.

More evidence can be provided by a patient's basal body temperature – the temperature taken immediately upon waking, before getting out of bed. Basal temperature is usually lower than normal in hypothyroid patients. In a woman who isn't pregnant, feverish, on progesterone therapy – or isn't at the point mid-cycle when she just ovulated – basal temperature should be around 98 degrees Fahrenheit. Severely hypothyroid patients often have a basal temperature in the low 97s or even in the 96s. I've seen a few even lower than 96. There aren't many other conditions that create low body temperature other than septic shock or environmental exposure to cold, so a low basal body temperature is very suggestive of low thyroid function. Dr. Broda Barnes routinely had his new patients measure their basal temperatures before seeing them to aid in the diagnosis and to show his patients objective evidence of low metabolic rates. And, of course, the patient's temp usually returns to normal when the patient is well replaced with thyroid. So, physicians, ask your patients if their body temperature usually runs low. And patients, track your basal temperature – you'll need a basal thermometer – and share that information with your doctor!

One other point about using cold hands to diagnose hypothyroidism: Estrogen-deficient women who are postmenopausal and not on hormone replacement tend to be hot all the time and hot to the touch, even if they are also hypothyroid. If one of these women has cold hands, they are likely hypothyroid.

Finally, an important detail about treatment: In most of my

patients who had cold extremities, felt cold all the time, or had a low basal temperature, I found that their symptoms responded best to the addition of T4 rather than T3.

REDUCED IMMUNITY

> *"If much or all of your life, you've been prone to get what has seemed to you to be more than a normal share of respiratory and other infections and those you get are generally severe and prolonged, you belong to a sizeable group of people. I've seen many such patients and I have belonged in the group myself."*

Those are the words of Broda Barnes in his 1976 book, *Hypothyroidism, the Unsuspected Illness,*[130] but they could just as easily have been my own words. Before I began taking thyroid hormone, I was plagued by frequent sinus infections every winter. It became so bad during one particularly persistent month-long infection that it resisted *all* the antibiotics that I could swallow. I ended up asking my friend Vesna, an otolaryngologist, for her help. I was feverish, miserable, and afraid that the pus that had set up residence in my maxillary sinuses was about to break through into my cerebral cavity and kill me. I was so sick I thought I was going to die.

Vesna had a fabulous Eastern European accent and a habit of calling everyone "Dahling." After growing up in a country taken over by Communists, she was a resourceful and ferocious woman of action with incredible survival skills. I trusted her completely. I vividly remember sitting in her exam chair in her office as she injected and stuffed my nose full of every "-caine" drug in her cabinet – Xylocaine, Procaine, Carbocaine – to prepare me for what came next. She then got out an instrument that looked exactly like my mother's old wooden-handled icepick and carefully pushed it through the back of my nose and the boney wall into my maxillary sinus. I felt pressure and could "hear" her instrument perforate the sinus wall as the vibrations conducted through the bones of my head to my ears, but otherwise, I felt no pain.

The next thing I knew, out came what seemed like gallons of horrid green slime, far worse than anything you may have seen on the

Nickelodeon Channel! I was thrilled to have survived this ordeal, glad to have that horrible green stuff released from my head, and within the next 12 hours, my temperature returned to normal, and I was miraculously cured! Vesna is my hero, and I am forever indebted to her for literally saving my life. I learned in my gynecology residency that pus needs to find a way out, and Vesna certainly helped that process along quite efficiently and effectively.

Since I have been on thyroid replacement, I no longer have recurrent and unrelenting sinus infections. Instead, I have an occasional minor bout with mild sinusitis. That's good because Vesna and her ice pick have retired, and no one out there could ever take her place!

Basic research confirms a positive effect of thyroid hormone on immune function. In a 1984 study published by Moley, Ohkawa, et al.,[131] hypothyroid rats and control rats were made septic via bowel ligation and puncture, and their immune responses were measured. They measured physiologic immune responses like oxygen consumption, hepatic blood flow, normal hyperglycemic response, and survival. They also studied hypothyroid rats that had their thyroid hormone replaced via daily injections of thyroxine. The researchers found that:

> *"The absence of thyroid hormone abolishes the hyperdynamic phase of sepsis and significantly increases mortality in sepsis, and thyroxine replacement following thyroidectomy prevents the increased mortality from sepsis."*

Are we surprised? No.

Broda Barnes devoted an entire chapter in his book to discussing how common it was for hypothyroid patients to have recurrent and frequent infections. He noted that these patients have more colds, sore throats, ear infections, boils, carbuncles, influenza, pneumonia, rheumatic fever, and even deaths due to infectious processes. Here is one of the cases he described in this book:

> *"A college boy who had a serious automobile accident in which several bones were fractured, developed osteomyelitis in a leg.*

> *Again, despite antibiotics, the infection kept recurring. His parents were hypothyroid and on thyroid therapy. The boy, too, was hypothyroid and I had placed him on thyroid therapy some years before. But, on this own, he had decided that he need not take thyroid and had stopped it about a year before the accident. The recurrent osteomyelitis brought him to his senses and he returned to thyroid therapy; not long afterward, the osteomyelitis was gone." (p. 98)*

In his second book, *The Riddle of Heart Attacks,*[132] Dr. Barnes demonstrated a strong correlation between mortality due to tuberculosis and hypothyroidism. Similarly, a 2016 study by Tan, Rajeswaran, Haddad, et al.[133] found from a review of 32,289 hospital charts that patients with hypothyroidism were 2.46 times more likely to develop an infection in a prosthetic joint compared to normal patients. "In addition, patients who developed PJI, [periprosthetic joint infections], demonstrated higher thyroid-stimulating hormone levels than those without."

Further, a quick review of the basic scientific literature reveals more evidence that supports the idea that hypothyroidism results in a sluggish immune response. A study in 1991 by Liu and Ng[134] reports that phagocytosis by macrophages – the ability of immune cells to consume and destroy infectious agents – was reduced in rats treated with a drug that reduces thyroid function. Then in 2009, Hodkinson, Simpson, Beattie, et al.[135] measured various immune cells, lymphocytes, activated monocytes, etc., and found that even "within normal physiological ranges," the amount of thyroid hormone present was positively associated with the number of immune cells present in 93 healthy individuals. Several years later, Papaioannou, Michelis, et al.[136] demonstrated that lymphocyte activation and blastogenesis – the production of more immune cells – in response to a stimulant was reduced in hypothyroid patients compared to normal controls. These findings were confirmed the same year in a study[137] by De Vito, Incerpi, et al. The bottom line is that our immune systems become sluggish when thyroid function is reduced.

During my decades of treating hypothyroid patients, I saw dozens of cases where fixing a thyroid deficiency improved a patient's ability to fight off infections. For example, I saw a patient years ago who had almost monthly and very distressing outbreaks of genital herpes. After replacing her thyroid adequately, she rarely had outbreaks at all. She was able to stop taking a daily dose of the antiviral drug Valtrex. This also happens with cold sores.

Other patients of mine, plagued by frequent urinary tract infections, were relieved of that problem once their thyroid problems were addressed. And like me, many of my patients had significantly fewer sinus and respiratory infections after starting thyroid replacement. I even noticed a reduction in seasonal allergies in multiple patients after they began thyroid replacement. Stimulating patients' immune systems with thyroid replacement was a great way to make patients' health a lot less complicated and easier to maintain!

THE DWINDLES

I learned about a condition called "the dwindles" during medical school and my residency. In a 1995 *Los Angeles Times* article entitled "Elderly Cope With 'The Dwindles,'"[138] Cassandra Burrell described the dwindles in this way:

> *"Reclusiveness, a lack of appetite, declining energy and some other ailments commonly associated with aging may be signs of a condition known as "the dwindles,' or, as doctors call it, 'failure to thrive.'"*

The dwindles can cause a dramatically reduced appetite. Elderly women with the dwindles, in fact, often stop eating entirely and don't do much except sleep. Eventually, they wither away as they succumb to one health complication after another. I'm not sure if there's even an ICD 10 code for the dwindles, but anyone who has ever seen nursing home patients knows exactly what I am talking about.

Having "the dwindles" is pretty much a death sentence since body systems like the skeletal system, the cardiovascular system, and the immune system don't work very well when no nutrition comes in. There's also no known cure for the dwindles. But suppose you could do something to give them back their appetite. You could get them a few more years of a hopefully good life by preventing the inevitable dwindles and potentially life-ending health complications. Often, the final coup de grace is a hip or pelvic fracture, which occurs at least in part due to a lack of appetite and poor nutritional status.

Doesn't this condition sound like Jenna, the little 12-year-old girl with gastroparesis and no appetite, who was nutrient deficient because her gut was asleep? Why not treat these women who have the dwindles with a bit of thyroid and see if we can stimulate them to eat?

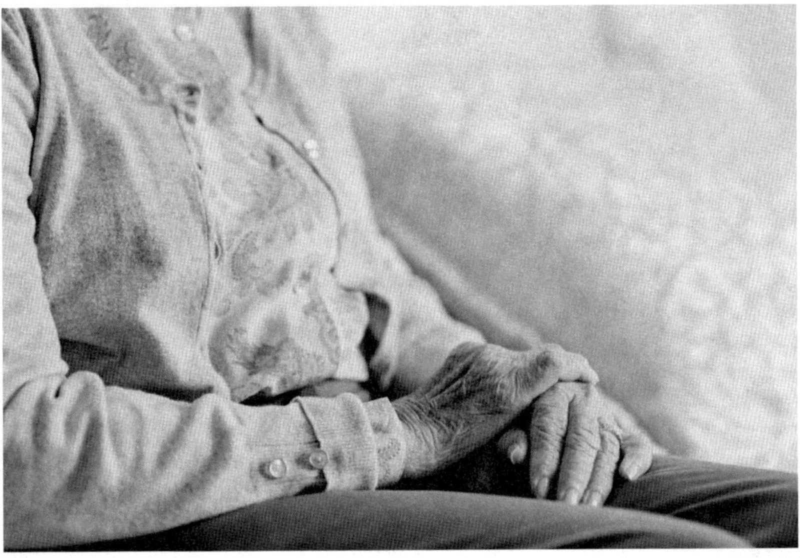

Years ago, I had the opportunity to do just that. I saw a previously spunky 91-year-old new patient who complained that she was tired, had little appetite, and lacked enthusiasm. She spent far too many hours sleeping. Her other doctors had written those symptoms off as usual for her age, but her daughter brought her in to see me because she thought I might be able to help her. Her daughter was my patient and had significantly benefited from thyroid replacement herself.

We started with a very small dose of thyroid and slowly increased, being very cautious not to overdose this elderly woman. Sure enough, she started feeling a lot better. Soon, her appetite was restored, and she started making jokes and enjoying her life again! I saw her until she was 99, and she never had any problems with her thyroid replacement. I'm so glad I could restore her capacity for joy and vitality during those precious final years of her life!

If I were a geriatrician or a doctor who treated patients in nursing homes, I certainly would want to give a trial of thyroid to every little old lady suffering from the dwindles. Obviously, great care needs to be taken with dosing, and the dose should go up *very* slowly, as I did with my 91-year-old patient. In her case, we had an excellent outcome. Since the outcome of this condition without treatment is universally quite grim, why not give it a try?

PART 3: PRACTICAL ASPECTS OF CLINICALLY-BASED THYROID DOSING

CHAPTER 14: HOW TO MEASURE OUTCOMES AND CHOOSE THYROID PRODUCTS

"Life is a series of adjustments. You can make changes along the way, but if you don't start moving forward, you'll never get anywhere!"
~ Kimora Lee Simmons

The best dose of thyroid hormone for each patient is the one that best relieves all of their symptoms and signs of hypothyroidism and, at the same time, is a dose that does no harm. That seems relatively straightforward, even if it's not part of the official practice guidelines. This chapter details my approach to determining the best possible dose for each woman with hypothyroidism.

GENERAL CONSIDERATIONS

The misguided goal of many endocrinologists and physicians today is to give a dose of thyroid hormone that achieves a TSH level in the current "normal range." Unfortunately, relieving symptoms and creating true wellness is no longer a key part of the equation.

I found that the doses of thyroid hormone that make patients clinically well and relieve symptoms vary all over the place, ranging from tiny amounts of less than 50 mg (½ grain) daily to more than 1000 mg (10 grains) of thyroid. That sounds like a lot, and it is, but remember that larger doses were commonly used before the TSH blood test was adopted as a surrogate marker for clinical wellness.

During my many years of practice, I found that to reach clinical wellness, most patients need doses somewhere in the middle of that range. The distribution of optimal doses seems to be in a bell-shaped curve, with most patients falling in the middle and a much smaller number at both ends.

Remember, nearly *all* patients with hypothyroidism will have a "normal" TSH level that falls within the reference range when taking a small dose of thyroid medication, usually ranging from 30 to 90 mg (½ to 1 ½ grains) of NDT (or 50 to 150 mcg of levothyroxine). This explains why patients who are treated until the TSH is normal are *usually* not clinically well and still have all the symptoms that they had before treatment was started. And that's why so many of them end up frustrated and seeking a different approach.

To optimally serve patients, physicians must first acknowledge that the needs of each patient are unique. In addition, health care providers need to be willing to work with patients to find the exact dose of the right thyroid medication to resolve that patient's symptoms.

I'll be straight with you. There is no easy, fool-proof way to do this. The best dose isn't related to a patient's weight, age, duration of treatment, or even the severity of their symptoms. The only way to find the best dose for each patient is to start with a small amount and carefully titrate the dose upward, step by step until the symptoms disappear.

I usually started patients on a small dose, around 30 mg (½ grain) of NDT (or 50 mcg of levothyroxine), once or twice a day. I would increase that dose by about 30 mg (½ grain) of NDT (or 50 mcg of T4) every two to four weeks. What is crucial to this treatment method is that both practitioner and patient must stay vigilant to watch for, recognize, and appropriately respond to any signs or symptoms of overdose. This is important both during the period when the dosage is being adjusted and after, when the patient reaches an optimal dose.

Why is it essential to put so much emphasis on watching for overdose? In practice, I found that the best dose to relieve the most stubborn symptoms was almost always slightly below the dose that would overmedicate the patient.

Some goals – for example, increasing energy, body temperature, and resolution of constipation – were achievable, even when the dose was not optimal. But when weight loss or warming cold hands and feet is a goal, the dose needs to be near perfect – which means an amount just shy of overmedication.

It usually takes a near-perfect amount of thyroid to raise the metabolic rate enough to generate enough warmth to heat the hands and feet. I often told my patients not to expect any weight loss until their feet were warm to the touch. The dose that resolves those symptoms is usually the patient's optimal dose.

A caveat: There are always exceptions. The key to success is for both physician and patient to be constantly observant, cautious, and open-minded when determining the best dose.

WHAT SHOULD BE THE GOAL OF THERAPY: CLINICAL WELLNESS OR NORMAL LABS?

Sir William Osler said, "The greater the ignorance, the greater the dogmatism." And dogmatism is rampant in the conventional treatment of hypothyroidism.

Endocrinologists have been taught that optimal thyroid doses can be calculated based on their patient's weight. Consequently, they tend to give 1.6 mcg of T4 per kg of the patient's weight. This calculation usually leads to a dose of about 100 mcg, give or take 50 mcg, given as a once-a-day morning dose on an empty stomach. Then the endocrinologist makes minor adjustments to the dose every six weeks or so, with follow-up lab tests each time to see if that particular dose is the correct dose to achieve normal lab results. That allows them to eventually reach a "normal" TSH level, which is their ultimate goal.

The problem is that most thyroid patients aren't satisfied with this approach because many – if not most of them – remain unwell, and most of their symptoms persist even after the TSH is normalized. For this reason, I think we should essentially ignore that arbitrary weight-based calculation of dosage and the TSH monitoring method when determining a patient's optimal dose of thyroid hormone. I know I'm being redundant, and the endocrinology world thinks these words are nothing short of heresy, but this is the book's most important message.

I'm not alone. Some others hold the same perspective, even though it puts us in conflict with conventional medicine and their Big Pharma friends, who enjoy financial benefits when hypothyroidism is inadequately diagnosed and treated. For example, Matvey Brokhin, Sara Danzi, and Irwin Klein wrote in their 2019 article in *Frontiers in Endocrinology*:[139] "Recent studies identify a significant number of hypothyroid patients who express dissatisfaction with their therapy." They blamed their dissatisfaction on the difficulty that physicians have in detecting hypothyroidism and inadequately treating it when it's eventually diagnosed. They rightly stated that measurement of the TSH "may not be a reliable measure of thyroid hormone in action in individual patients," relating that problem to the presence of "thyroid hormone resistance," among other things. In these cases, they suggested:

> *"It would be useful to have an additional quantitative clinical measure that both directly and indirectly reflects the cellular action of thyroid hormone and could be used clinically to aid in diagnosis and treatment."*

To address this deficiency, they proposed using a list of "clinically relevant hypothyroid symptoms" commonly present in patients with thyroid disease as "a tool that could help clinicians to assess adequacy of LT4 treatment." They also proposed a questionnaire asking patients to rate ten physical symptoms of thyroid disease, including "dry skin, fatigue, weight gain, cold intolerance, constipation, muscle stiffness, puffiness, early awakening, memory loss, and feeling blue."

They add that "hypothyroid symptom scales have been previously developed and modified over the years to primarily aid in the diagnosis of hypothyroidism." For example, they refer to an article from 1969 by Billewicz et al.[140] that "described a diagnostic index that assessed the presence or absence of various signs and symptoms of hypothyroidism for the purpose of establishing a diagnosis of hypothyroidism." Interestingly, when compared to laboratory measures, they found that "the score correlated with FT4 and FT3, [but] it did not correlate with TSH, the gold standard for thyroid function testing."

Concerning Brokhin's proposed 2019 clinically relevant hypothyroid symptoms questionnaire, they found that:

> *"Using this tool, we have identified persistently symptomatic hypothyroid patients who subsequent to appropriate changes in levothyroxine dosages then showed improvement.... The hypothyroid symptom scale showed a statistically significant improvement in the sum of the signs and symptoms with the normalization of the subjects' thyroid function."*

Unfortunately, the improvements seen were somewhat limited because the researchers limited the amount that they increased the thyroid doses to doses that would maintain a TSH in the normal range. This is a bit perplexing since the point of their paper was to show that TSH is inadequate as a measure of hypothyroidism! Nonetheless, they did find improvements even with small dose increases – about 25 mcg of T4 on average – and also found additional improvements with the addition of T3. They concluded that:

> *"In the case of suspected inadequate thyroid hormone replacement, the clinician may opt for LT4 dose increase, change in LT4 formulation or the addition of liothyronine. The*

proposed hypothyroid symptom scale showed a statistically significant improvement in the subjects' thyroid function."

The National Academy of Hypothyroidism[141] was established about 10 years ago by a group of physicians who sought to improve understanding of diagnosis and treatment of hypothyroidism, disseminate new knowledge, and "implement change in 'standard' endocrinological dogma that has historically left the majority of patients misdiagnosed as euthyroid (normal thyroid) based on the use of inaccurate out dated 'standard' blood tests." Their website includes a number of articles concerning the inadequacy of using TSH as a measure of thyroid hormone function. Their 2012 review article, "How Accurate is TSH Testing?"[142] which impressively includes 118 references, explains that because the pituitary (where TSH is made) responds differently to circulating thyroid hormone than do the peripheral tissues:

> *"TSH isn't a reliable or sensitive marker of an individual's true thyroid status…TSH is, however, merely a marker of pituitary levels of T3 and not of T3 levels in any other part of the body… making the TSH a poor indicator of the body's overall thyroid status."*

Like the Brokhin article, they reference yet another article[143] that suggested using a clinical score of 14 common signs and symptoms of hypothyroidism to measure thyroid function. Like the Billewicz study from 1969, they:

> *"found that the clinical score and ankle reflex time correlated well with tissue thyroid effect but the TSH had no correlation with the tissue effect of thyroid hormone…. Making both the measurement of the reflex speed and clinical assessment a more accurate measurement of tissue thyroid effect than the TSH.*
>
> *Forgoing treatment based on a normal TSH without further assessment will result in the misdiagnosis or mismanagement of a large number of hypothyroid patients that may greatly benefit with treatment. Simply relying on a TSH to determine the thyroid status of a patient demonstrates a lack of understanding of thyroid physiology and isn't evidence-based medicine."*

The National Academy of Hypothyroidism authors also addressed the proverbial elephant in the room in their 2012 article, "Why Doesn't My Endocrinologist Know All of This?"[144]

Why are endocrinologists and physicians who comply with the TSH dogma so enamored by the idea that TSH measures thyroid function and should be used exclusively to diagnose and manage hypothyroidism? This article offered several important answers:

1. The typical consensus statements held up as a standard of care are considered "the poorest level of evidence" because they typically ignore any new information and findings in the medical literature. Shockingly, "even the strongest (Class 1) recommendations, which are considered medical dogma [and] cited as a legal standard, often go unquestioned as medical fact, [and]were only supported by high-quality evidence 19% of the time and not revised based on new evidence."
2. The medical establishment is resistant to new ideas, and even then, physicians – notorious for not keeping up with the latest medical research – are painfully slow to adopt any new recommendations.
3. Sidney Smith, MD, the former president of the American Heart Association, said that doctors often feel the best medicine is what they've been doing and thinking for years. They discount new research because "it isn't what they have been taught or practiced, and they refuse to admit that what they have been doing or thinking for many years is not the best medicine."
4. The National Institute of Medicine has found that "The lag between the discovery of more effective forms of treatment and their incorporation into routine patient care averages 17 years."
5. Most physicians meet their continuing medical education (CME) requirements by going to one conference a year – sponsored by pharmaceutical companies and held at a luxury vacation destination. As a result, "groundbreaking research that goes against the status quo and does not support the drug industry receives little attention."

The article concluded with what I consider one of the most important paragraphs you can read about hypothyroidism:

> *"Evidence-based medicine involves the synthesis of all available data when comparing therapeutic options for patients. Evidence-based medicine does not mean that data should be ignored until a randomized controlled trial of a particular size and duration is completed... The best doctors who truly practice evidence-based medicine and not merely the perception of such will not rely on consensus statements to best provide their patients. Instead of relying on old dogma, the best physicians will seek out and translate both the basic science results and clinical outcomes to decide on the safest, most efficacious treatment of their patients. Further, the best physicians will continually assess the current available data to decide which therapies are likely to carry the greatest benefits for patients and involve the lowest risks."*

Indeed, as Daniel Boorstin, former librarian to Congress, famously said,[145] "The greatest obstacle to discovering the shape of the earth, the continents, and the oceans was not ignorance, but the illusion of knowledge." And in the field of hypothyroidism diagnosis and treatment, there is no greater illusion of knowledge than the belief that TSH measures thyroid function!

MEASURE FUNCTION – NOT AMOUNT – OF THYROID!

Before starting any hypothyroid patient on thyroid replacement, I always explained what thyroid does in the body and how it controls metabolism or metabolic rate. I might say, "It's like a computer operating system for your body; it drives all the programs in your body; it tells each part of your body what to do and at what rate to do it." Or "It's like your thermostat or your accelerator pedal in your car. It determines how fast your body uses fuel to produce heat and energy."

Then I'd ask them if they know of any single test that can measure whether or not their computer's operating system is working correctly. Is it adequate to look into the computer system information to see that "Windows" is present in the computer? Does that tell whether or not the operating system is working properly to run all the programs on the computer? Of course not! To see if Windows is working properly, you need to test all the programs in the computer that it drives. Is the screen working properly? Is there sound? Does the mouse move the cursor? Can you access the internet? Can you upload or download? Does Word work correctly?

Similarly, to measure thyroid function, you can't just measure whether enough thyroid hormone – the TSH, free T3, free T4, etc. – is present in the bloodstream. And that's *all* the lab tests do. Doing lab tests to measure thyroid function is like looking in your computer's system information to see if Windows is loaded on your computer. Yes, it's there. But that doesn't tell you anything about whether Windows is functioning correctly, any more than the TSH values tell you about thyroid hormone function. As we discussed earlier, blood tests don't measure metabolism – the function of thyroid. In fact, there isn't a blood test in existence that can directly measure metabolism. As a result, we need an alternative, and that's where clinical assessment comes in.

THE TYRANNY OF THE TSH!

The pituitary gland, which makes TSH, can't differentiate between functional and non-functional thyroid hormones. So, it measures and reacts to the total amount of thyroid in the bloodstream, both functional and non-functional. The pituitary also usually thinks there is too much thyroid present when a patient is, in fact, well replaced. The same is true when measuring free T3 and free T4 since they also measure a total amount of hormone and can't identify how much of that hormone is functional. (It's like the IRS taxing your total income instead of your adjusted gross income. You'll always end up paying more and ending up with less!) No blood test can differentiate functional from nonfunctional thyroid hormone, so efforts to manage thyroid hormone replacement by lab test alone almost always yield the wrong answer.

When thyroid hormone is being properly and fully replaced, it will usually make other doctors uncomfortable. This is unavoidable. My solution? Before starting treatment, I always warned a patient that her other doctors *would likely* have an issue with her thyroid treatment. And the best way to avoid this discomfort is for her to refuse to allow other doctors to do thyroid tests or review any thyroid test results. After all, if a doctor isn't managing the patient's thyroid replacement, there's no reason for that doctor to order thyroid lab tests.

Though I was happy to have my patients' other doctors see and clinically evaluate them while they were on thyroid; take a history, do a physical exam, check vital signs, do an EKG, etc., I encouraged my patients to tell their other physicians that they did *not* give them permission to perform thyroid labs. But this was often easier said than done, to put it mildly! These days, "having a physical" usually involves a primary care provider ordering dozens of random lab tests before they even talk to or see a patient. The lab results are posted on the patient's online portal for the patient to review and analyze on their own or with the help of the internet, friends, or family. Physicians rarely explain the results, and many offer no real clinical evaluation. Without the battery of random tests, these physicians could hardly justify their submission of an ICD 10 code for having done a "physical." Modern-day doctors have been trained to depend on labs and to consider a battery of lab tests as a sacred part of every patient encounter.

Despite my advice, patients sometimes forgot, or their requests were ignored. Inevitably, other doctors would order labs anyway, expressing concern about the patient's TSH levels. Some of those doctors seemed to think that they alone knew what was best for their patients. And rather than contacting me to discuss the treatment plan, these doctors would conclude that our unfamiliar treatment was wrong, and they had no qualms about saying that to our mutual patients – often in a very disparaging and dogmatic way. This puts my patients in a difficult position, trapped between two competing approaches. On one side was me, with the goal of clinical wellness. On the other side was a doctor whose goal was strict compliance with standard dogma. The poor patients ended up stuck in the middle.

And then, when the TSH results showed a suppressed thyroid – despite the patient being completely well with absolutely no clinical evidence of thyroid overdose – these physicians authoritatively declared that my patient was overdosed. Some of them went on a campaign to scare the patient with worst-case scenarios about hyperthyroidism, even though we were carefully and constantly monitoring the patient for signs of overdose, and the patient wasn't experiencing any of those symptoms. For example, they would declare that the patient was losing bone without even bothering to look at the results of the patient's serial bone density tests that showed no bone loss. Usually, that physician would then advise the patient to stop taking the thyroid until they could establish a new and much lower dose based solely on lab tests.

This situation, repeated many times during my years in practice, was frightening for patients. Out of fear, some complied, even though the only thing that wasn't normal was their TSH level. And sadly, when a patient who is clinically well stops or even reduces the dose of thyroid hormone, the benefits are lost.

I remember one patient who saw an endocrinologist. He never checked her blood pressure or weight and didn't do a physical exam. He simply looked at her TSH level, declared that she was overmedicated, and insisted that she lower her dose. That is considered "good medicine" these days, and frankly, it's disheartening. My late friend Dr. Gordon Skinner summed up this experience on page 21 of his 2003 book:[146]

> *"An Endocrinologist pronounces – often with some irritation – that the patient is definitely not hypothyroid and spouts cock about evidence-based-medicine, having omitted to take the patient's pulse or temperature or even listen to the woman."*

NATURAL DESICCATED THYROID (T4 +T3)

As we discussed much earlier, the only thyroid product available to doctors when thyroid treatment first became commonplace was natural desiccated thyroid, aka Armour Thyroid. That product is still on the market, though it has changed hands several times. In addition, we currently also have NP Thyroid made by Acella

THYROID HORMONE REPLACEMENT DRUGS

Natural Desiccated Thyroid (NDT) Tablets
(Porcine thyroid with both T4 and T3)
- Armour Thyroid (brand)
- NP Thyroid (brand/generic)
- Nature-Throid (brand)
- WP Thyroid (brand)
- Westhroid (brand))

Synthetic T3 / Liothyronine Tablets
- Cytomel (brand)
- Liothyronine (generic)

Compounded Thyroid Hormone Replacement Capsules
- Compounded Levothyroxine (T4)
- Compounded Liothyronine (T3)
- Compounded Sustained-Release (SR) Liothyronine (SR-T3)
- Compounded Thyroid USP (Natural Desiccated Thyroid/NDT)
- Compounded Custom Combination of T4, T3/SR-T3, and/or NDT

Synthetic T4 / Levothyroxine Tablets
- Synthroid (brand)
- Levoxyl (brand)
- Unithroid (brand)
- Euthyrox (brand)
- Levothyroxine (generic)

Synthetic T4 / Levothyroxine Liquid
- Tirosint (liquid gel capsules)
- Tirosint-SOL (oral solution in ampules)

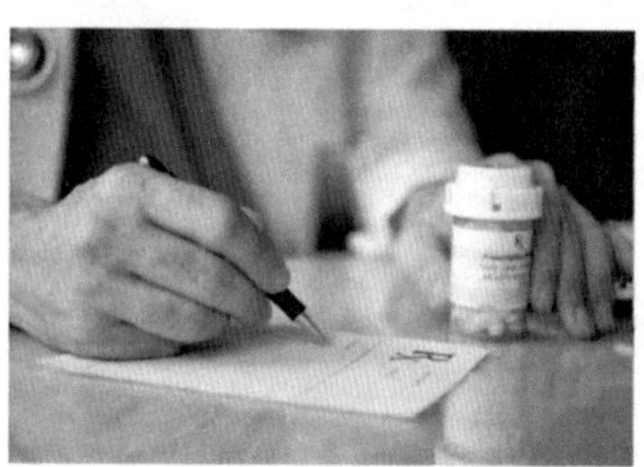

Pharmaceuticals, which is a different and less expensive brand of natural desiccated thyroid that happens to be gluten-free. Recently, we also had Nature-Throid and Westhroid, both made by a small American company called RLC Labs, but it seems that for at least the time being, those products are no longer available. We can also have natural desiccated thyroid compounded at compounding pharmacies. Compounded NDT is beneficial for patients who need a unique dose or when they need to avoid certain allergenic fillers found in the other products. Of course, NDT isn't usually an option for someone with a pork allergy, although I did have one patient with a pork allergy who tolerated it without a problem.

Since the thyroid gland of a pig isn't man-made but occurs naturally, NDT drugs contain *all* of the components that one finds naturally in a pig's thyroid gland. That would include T3 and T4, and other thyroid hormones and precursor compounds. I used natural desiccated thyroid when I wanted to give my patient some T3 and often mixed it with a straight T4 product. That way, the T3/T4 ratio more closely reflects that of a human (where there is relatively more T4 and less T3 than what is found in a pig's thyroid gland.). Pharmacies will often dispense NP Thyroid as if it were generic, but in reality, it's basically a less expensive brand of natural desiccated thyroid.

CYTOMEL (LIOTHYRONINE/T3)

The other T3 product we have in our toolbox is Cytomel, the only straight synthetic T3 (liothyronine) brand available. As one would expect, since it's the only branded T3 product, it's generally quite expensive. Generic liothyronine is also available, but in my experience, there can be quite a lot of potency variation with generic T3 products. That can create problems because pure T3 is potent and short-acting from the onset, so minimal changes in potency or absorption have a dramatic effect clinically. A patient might be doing ok on a specific dose of Cytomel. Still, when her pharmacy inevitably plays the old bait and switch with her and gives her a generic T3 – often without informing the patient of such a switch – she may suddenly become significantly overdosed or underdosed.

Again, T3 is very short acting. It goes in quickly and comes out just as quickly. Some patients get a "buzz" from it about an hour after they take it, as the serum level is peaking. And then, later in the day, the effect seems to vanish. At most, T3 has about six to eight hours of effectiveness in the typical patient, even if it's compounded as a "long-acting" or sustained-release product. Therefore, it needs to be prescribed at least twice a day, sometimes even more frequently. Most endocrinologists seem to be aware of this problem with T3, and those who use it often prescribe it in two doses a day when they do prescribe it.

Some "experts" in the thyroid community (I won't bother to list them here) suggest that patients should be given only T3 multiple times a day, and T4 should not be prescribed because patients "can't convert T4 to T3" and "T3 is the active form of thyroid," or T4 "creates too much reverse T3." I disagree. Most of my patients found a mixture of T3 and T4 to work best – usually heavy on the T4 side. T4's effect is more constant and seems to be quite a bit "softer" – with fewer sharp highs and no sharp lows—compared to T3. That said, I did work with several patients on a T3-only treatment. One took six tiny doses of T3 every day. But it's cumbersome to take doses of a short-acting product many times a day just to maintain effectiveness.

As for people who are supposedly "unable to convert T4 to T3," I have some questions.

1. How do you know you can't convert T4 to T3?
2. Have you determined that based on laboratory measurements of free T3 and free T4?
3. How do you know that your lab results are measuring the functions of T3 and T4? (Hint: They don't!)

In my experience, giving patients T4 frequently improved symptoms that seem dependent on T3, such as constipation or dry skin. And ultimately, I found that for many patients, T4 did indeed improve T3 function – even if no T3 was prescribed. I also saw patients taking only T4 who were on too much and developed symptoms of overdose usually associated with too much T3. As Robin Thicke and Pharrell sang[147] in their 2013 hit song, there are definitely "blurred lines" between T4 and T3!

This is why treating patients with a defined amount of T3 and T4 to normalize free T3 and T4 levels makes no sense to me. I believe it's best just to try what you think might work and assess the clinical result. If the results aren't optimal, the dose should be adjusted. If a woman needs more thyroid – but increasing T3 or NDT will provide too much T3 effect – then increase straight T4 instead. Simple.

SYNTHROID AND THE OTHER LEVOTHYROXINE DRUGS

Several branded T4 (levothyroxine) products are currently available. Synthroid is the best known and is one of the most expensive of these drugs and has been on the market the longest. They also have the most visible and aggressive sales force. Many endocrinologists seem to believe that Synthroid is the "gold standard" thyroid product and, as a result, it's the only thyroid drug that they prescribe. It's a small round pill that tastes somewhat sweet because it contains confectioners' sugar. It also contains lactose, corn starch, and a small amount of gluten. Levoxyl is another brand of T4. This tablet comes in the shape of a bow tie, is relatively soft, and quickly disintegrates when swallowed. Consequently, the manufacturer of Levoxyl recommends you drink a full 8-ounce glass of water when taking Levoxyl pills. The tablets are easy to break in half with your fingers.

Unithroid is another round tablet. It's gluten-free, and the manufacturer offers generous discount programs. I'm on that product currently. The Unithroid company also tries very hard to keep the price of Unithroid very affordable. Not surprisingly, it's growing in popularity. Another drug, Euthyrox, is free of gluten, lactose, and dyes and came to the US market from Europe. Made by Merck, this T4 pill is unique in that it has very few excipients and fillers and is dispensed in individual blister packs, which protects the medication from moisture and light.

Finally, there's also a liquid form of T4. Tirosint brand levothyroxine comes as a liquid in a gel capsule. Tirosint-SOL is a liquid that comes in a small single-dose ampule. Tirosint's claim to fame is that it contains no dyes, and its only ingredients are levothyroxine, water, gelatin, and glycerin. Tirosint was first released as a specialty T4 for patients with allergies and absorption problems, but it's become popular with patients who don't do well on traditional T4 tablets. Tirosint can be quite pricey, and getting it filled at a local pharmacy can be a challenge in terms of pre-authorization requirements and high prices. The manufacturer offers the Tirosint Direct mail program, which takes care of the preauthorization problems and dispenses Tirosint and Tirosint-SOL at a deep discount. (Tirosint does not offer a 300 mcg dose.)

In addition to the branded T4 tablets and the Tirosint products, there are also many manufacturers distributing generic T4 tablets. Like all generics, the challenge is that all the different fillers affect absorption rates. And that will affect the potency of the product. Absorption will also be affected by whether the pill is taken with food or on an empty stomach.

These variations in the potency of generics are a big problem for the conventional medical world since they rely almost exclusively on the TSH test result. TSH varies logarithmically with the dose, particularly around the 100-mcg dose range, so tiny changes in thyroid dose or potency can yield dramatic shifts in the TSH. As a result, once a patient is on the "perfect dose" of a specific thyroid drug that delivers the "perfect" TSH, doctors who live and die by TSH values *really* don't like any changes in the treatment regimen. I believe this is why doctors insist on brand-name products as a rule and why patients are told to take their pills away from food since food can slightly interfere with the absorption of thyroid pills and cause shifts in the TSH level.

In contrast, if the goal is simply clinical wellness, those slight variations in potency with food or changes in the product brand are generally not that noticeable. That's why I am not a stickler for branded products, and I encourage my patients to take their second dose with lunch because it's easier to remember than taking an afternoon dose "on an empty stomach." Finally, it's preferable to stick with the same product if you can, but if it requires you to spend tons of money to do such, I would find a different product.

Here's an interesting fact about levothyroxine: As of September 2019, levothyroxine (generic T4) held the coveted position of being the most commonly prescribed pharmaceutical product in the US, and it was in that position for several years.[148] What is most interesting about this is that 8 of the 9 runner-up drugs are used to treat common symptoms of hypothyroidism that often persist when the thyroid replacement dosage is inadequate! For example,

Lisinopril, Amlodipine, Metoprolol, and Losartan are all used to treat high blood pressure. Atorvastatin and Simvastatin are used to treat high cholesterol, and Metformin is used to treat metabolic syndrome. Imagine how much money we could save by giving adequate thyroid doses to hypothyroid patients. We could avoid much of the need for all those other bestselling drugs!!

Sadly, I suspect that too many people in the medical/pharmaceutical industry – especially the ones who teach us to worship the TSH – perhaps do realize that little fact…and because all those drugs are so profitable, they would much prefer that we continue to underdose our patients with thyroid, thereby creating the need to supplement with all these other top-selling drugs. And the best way to assure that patients will continue to need all those drugs is to vigorously and dogmatically advocate for a "normal TSH" to be the goal of our therapy, which causes us to underdose our hypothyroid patients. I hope I'm wrong, but I fear I'm not.

COMPOUNDED THYROID DRUGS

Some patients must avoid certain fillers or need a unique (usually tiny) dose. I typically recommended specially compounded thyroid products, either a particular drug or several mixed together for those women. For example, I had a long-term patient who had multiple food and filler allergies and could not take any of the already manufactured products. In addition, when we started her on thyroid, she was exquisitely sensitive to even the smallest doses available. We, therefore, had hypoallergenic capsules made of tiny quantities of T4 and T3 separately, each mixed with a particular type of very pure salt (NaCl) as the only filler. Each capsule was just a few micrograms of thyroid. We used those T3 and T4 capsules as building blocks to gradually fine-tune and titrate her dose upward until we found the dose that resolved her symptoms. It was helpful that she had been an accomplished research scientist and was exceptionally skillful at keeping these tiny doses straight and carefully observing her clinical results.

I was very thankful to have good compounding pharmacists who made these products, particularly when tiny doses were needed. It's crucial to have that flexibility. Of course, you can also have natural desiccated thyroid capsules compounded if you need to, or you could have NDT mixed with T4 or with T3 if you like. I preferred to titrate with individual products when we were initially finding the best dose. And then, you can mix products into single capsules once you have determined the best ratio of T3 and T4.

CHAPTER 15: HOW TO FIND THE BEST DOSE

"To control your hormones is to control your life."
Barry Sears, MD

So how do we proceed with finding our patient's best dose of thyroid? What else do we need to know about thyroid dosing – specifically about the timing of dosing and the process of adjusting the dose up and down, known as titration? I've included some specific timing and titration guidelines in this chapter.

BASIC REQUIREMENTS FOR DOSE TITRATION

Finding the optimal dose of thyroid hormone for each patient requires careful titration of the dose, using the patient's clinical wellness as the goal. This is the original, old-fashioned way of finding the optimal dose, and in most cases, this method leads to a very happy and healthy patient. However, it does take some work on both the physician's and patient's part.

There are two main issues/requirements for this approach to be successful. The first is that in the process of finding the optimal dose, some patients may get too much thyroid hormone, which can cause symptoms of hyperthyroidism. This can easily be remedied by constantly monitoring for any signs that the dose is excessive and immediately reducing the dose. Since the body responds quite rapidly to changes in hormone levels, this approach is very effective and quickly resolves any symptoms of overmedication that may occur. Of course, this requires a compliant and motivated patient who is willing to monitor their body's functions daily for any signs of overdose and who will then notify their physician. I can't stress enough how vitally important this part is.

The second issue is that the dose that relieves all of a patient's symptoms will almost always yield a completely suppressed TSH that is close to or equal to 0. As I've discussed earlier in the book, the TSH becomes suppressed because it's measuring both the active thyroid that is affecting cellular function plus the patient's own inadequately functioning thyroid hormone. The result is that the TSH becomes suppressed early and falsely suggests that there is too much thyroid hormone.

This is no problem for someone who understands exactly what the TSH is measuring and what it is not measuring. But for most conventionally trained physicians, a suppressed TSH will make them *very* uncomfortable, as they will conclude that a suppressed TSH is evidence of overdosage. So, as we already discussed, this process requires the treating physician to understand that the goal of therapy goal is *not* a perfect TSH. Instead, normal thyroid *function* is the goal. Rarely do both exist simultaneously, so you need to choose one or the other. And in my experience, most patients choose wellness.

FIRST, DEFINE YOUR GOALS

After we've discussed the reasons for using clinical findings as opposed to laboratory tests to measure outcomes, and I'm satisfied that my patient understands the importance of that differentiation and is willing to do the necessary self-monitoring, the next step was to clearly define our desired outcome. Specifically, what individual symptoms do we want to correct?

I find that it's constructive to write out a list of the specific symptoms that have been bothering each patient and give a copy of that list to the patient, so the therapy goals are clearly defined at the onset. My list is very similar to the symptom lists offered by

Brokhin,[149] Billewicz,[150] and Zulewski[151] that we discussed earlier. The difference is that my list is unique to each patient and lists her particular symptoms. We'd draft the list together at the first visit and then use it later to see how many of the symptoms are resolved with our chosen therapy. I considered it a success when a patient enjoyed a 90% resolution of the symptoms on the list.

Below is a copy of the triplicate form that I used to list those individual symptoms as goalposts so that both the patient and I could remember what we were trying to accomplish. This list was also used as a symptom inventory checklist at follow-up visits to make sure that we have resolved (or at least improved) as many of the patient's symptoms as possible. One copy was given to the patient at the initial visit, one copy went into the chart notes for that day, and the other was saved for follow-up visits after the patient reached her optimal dose.

Donna Hurlock, MD

Phone:555-555-5555

****Please notify me of any new problems****

Clinical Goals and Doses for JANE DOE **Date** JUNE 1

GOALS	BETTER	SAME

AM DOSE	LUNCH DOSE	TAKE FOR

Please follow schedule as written. Do not alter it. Only go as high as you need to feel well. Do not exceed the dose that makes you well. Report any problems to us by fax or email with the title "Thyroid Status Report."

Followup visit due: ______________

As I mentioned earlier in the book, I also asked every new patient to review my general symptoms checklist below, check off her particular symptoms, indicate whether each symptom was mild, moderate, or severe, and bring that to our first consultation. We would use that general list as a springboard to create her personal form for guiding goals and dosage titration. Here again is my hypothyroidism/low thyroid symptom checklist.

Donna Hurlock, MD

HYPOTHYROIDISM/LOW THYROID SYMPTOMS CHECKLIST

Name ______________________ Date ____________

	Mild	Moderate	Severe
Fatigue	______	______	______
Weight gain	______	______	______
Depression	______	______	______
Anxiety	______	______	______
Memory Issues	______	______	______
Focus Issues (ADHD)	______	______	______
Migraines	______	______	______
Poor Sleep	______	______	______
Cold Intolerance	______	______	______
Heat Intolerance	______	______	______
Low Body Temperature	______	______	______
Hot Flashes	______	______	______
Cold Hands/Feet	______	______	______
Dry/Itchy Skin	______	______	______
Dry Eyes	______	______	______
Hair Loss	______	______	______
Water Retention	______	______	______
High Blood Pressure	______	______	______
Cravings	______	______	______
Constipation	______	______	______
High Cholesterol	______	______	______
Nasty Periods	______	______	______
Irregular Periods	______	______	______
Fertility Issues	______	______	______
No Sex Drive	______	______	______
Achy Joints	______	______	______
Achy Muscles	______	______	______
Tingling	______	______	______
Sensitive to Medicines	______	______	______
Sensitive to Coffee	______	______	______
______________	______	______	______
______________	______	______	______
______________	______	______	______

In addition to recording the patient's most bothersome symptoms on her goal list, I usually added the goal of keeping the resting evening pulse less than 85 to remind the patient each time she looks at her form to check her pulse every evening. Then a copy of that triplicate form was given to the patient as a reference during her dose titration process.

TWICE A DAY IS USUALLY OPTIMAL

Having done thyroid dose titration with thousands of patients over the last two decades, I strongly prefer twice-a-day dosing. When patients take all their thyroid medication in the morning, the effect of the morning dose seems to be gone by mid-afternoon. A second dose is needed to get through the rest of the day.

The first dose should be taken upon waking, with or without breakfast. I recommend taking the second dose four to six hours later, usually with lunch. I usually encouraged my patients to set their cell phone alarm for lunchtime to remind them to take their second pill. Why do I recommend the second dose, specifically with lunch? Mainly because it's easier to remember medications when you tie them to a meal. When patients try to find the right time to take the second dose on an empty stomach and timed separately from lunch, they invariably miss doses or stop taking a mid-day dose entirely and start taking both doses in the morning.

Taking the entire daily dose in the morning often causes hyperthyroidism symptoms by mid-morning, and then by mid-afternoon, patients are exhausted and desperate for a nap. Feeling especially tired, many women will also reach for sugary snacks, soda, or caffeine drinks for energy to get through the afternoon. Since weight loss is a common goal for many women with hypothyroidism, sugary and calorie-rich "pick-me-up snacks" are clearly counterproductive.

Another benefit of taking two daily doses is that the second dose gives women enough thyroid hormone to last well into the evening. This can help women stay asleep rather than waking up at 3 a.m., the classic mid-sleep witching hour for hypothyroid patients. I always asked my patients if they woke up at 3 a.m., and it's incredible how many hypothyroid patients said they did. This includes those patients who were already on thyroid hormone but only taking an early morning dose.

In addition to better energy in the afternoons and evenings, two daily doses also frequently resulted in more energy when waking up in the morning.

Finally, dosing twice a day helped patients burn calories for more than just eight or ten hours each day, sometimes resulting in some weight loss. I often encouraged my patients to think of the lunch dose as their *diet pill* to help motivate them to take it consistently.

One caveat: Patients shouldn't take the second dose too late in the day. If taken after work or around dinner time, women will likely reach peak energy around bedtime, which can play havoc with the ability to fall asleep. I did, however, have several patients who took their entire thyroid medication dose at bedtime and seemed to do fine with it and woke up rested. I saw no reason to argue with success in those few cases.

Occasionally, I gave a small amount of thyroid hormone at bedtime to help my patients stay asleep through the night and not wake up at 3 a.m. Remember, sleep is an active process and requires some energy expenditure to sleep efficiently. Usually, I would try about 25 mcg of T4 at bedtime. To be honest, sometimes it worked, and sometimes it didn't. But if a bit of T4 at bedtime improves sleep, I think it's better than taking a sleep aid like Ambien or Lunesta regularly. I found that a bedtime dose was rarely needed in most cases if the noontime dose was adequate.

It's important to remember that a century ago, thyroid hormone used to be given three times a day. Doctors in those days paid attention to their patient's clinical response to thyroid replacement and understood normal human physiology. They carefully adjusted the thyroid hormone replacement dose to optimize clinical benefits for their patients throughout the day and night. They didn't have lab tests to substitute for clinical assessment. Of course, these days, the emphasis is on TSH values, which tells us next to nothing about the effect of replacement thyroid on symptoms. Clinical outcome information has become simply irrelevant.

Spreading out the dose during the day helps avoid the highs and the lows that occur with once-a-day dosing. We need to, however, look beyond the TSH values, and appreciate the impact that the timing of dosing has on metabolism.

START LOW AND GO SLOW

Once the patient's goals were identified and listed, the next step was finding the optimal dose that eliminated most or all of the patient's symptoms without creating any new problems. Unless the patient was already on thyroid hormone from another physician or had a history of taking thyroid in the past, I usually started patients on ½ grain of thyroid (either 30 mg of NDT or 50 mcg of T4) upon waking and ½ grain (either NDT or T4) again at lunchtime. If the patient had significant problems with constipation, indigestion, low appetite, dry skin, dry eyes, hair loss, etc. – all symptoms of T3 deficiency – I would definitely start with some natural desiccated thyroid alone or perhaps mixed with some T4.

For example, the first dose might be NP Thyroid 30 mg (½ grain) upon waking with 50 mcg of T4 at noon. I found that most patients didn't do as well on straight natural desiccated thyroid, particularly if they ended up on a relatively large dose. Over time, the T3 was too overstimulating, especially if higher overall doses were needed.

If the patient's problems were primarily related to being cold and tired, and perhaps her pulse was low, I'd start her on T4 – for example, 50 mcg of T4 upon arising and another 50 mcg with lunch. Many patients do just fine on straight T4 without any natural desiccated thyroid. My current hypothyroidism treatment, for example, is only T4 and includes no natural desiccated thyroid. If that dose did not yield adequate benefit, then the dose was gradually increased every 2 to 4 weeks until most or all of the listed goals had been met, always being careful to avoid overmedication.

ASSESS RESULTS *CLINICALLY* AFTER EACH DOSE CHANGE

To find the best replacement, it's crucial to always pay attention to what is happening clinically after a change in dose and then adjust accordingly. This is important even when a woman's response to a particular dose of thyroid doesn't meet expectations. I always asked my patients, "Compared to the last dose, how has this symptom changed? Is it better, or is it worse?" The response usually allowed me to figure out if I was going in the right or wrong direction with dose adjustments. If a particular symptom was resolving, we were going in the right direction. If that symptom was getting worse, or a symptom of overdose occurred, we'd reverse direction. Over time, I'd have the patient adjust the dose every few weeks in small increments as we got closer to the best dose. When all the symptoms of hypothyroidism were resolved, with no adverse effects, we had reached our target: the correct dose!

Returning to my example, I always asked patients to report any new problems experienced during the first trial, which lasted around two weeks. Assuming no adverse effects have occurred, at the end of those two weeks, I'd ask her to review her list of symptoms and take an inventory of any changes she has noticed. She would do this at home and wasn't required to consult with me at that time unless she wanted to or was unsure what to do next.

If no changes in her symptoms and no harm were noticed, then we'd conclude that we were going in the right direction. The absence of adverse effects reassured us that we were going in the right direction.

If the patient noticed some small benefit from this first dose, that's even better. Let's say she felt around 10% better. Again, if there were no adverse effects, but the symptoms weren't fully resolved, I'd advise her to increase to the next dose. We usually increased the dose by ½ grain (30 mg of NDT or 50 mcg of T4) every two to three weeks, depending on the clinical effect. I would usually alternate the increases by increasing the morning dose and then increasing the lunchtime dose.

Therefore, after that first increase in the dose, the new dose would be 60 mg (1 grain) of natural desiccated thyroid in the morning, with 50 mcg of T4 with lunch. This process was continued until the low T3 symptoms were controlled. Once those symptoms were resolved, I would usually stop adding any additional natural desiccated thyroid since that can cause symptoms of excess T3 like jitteriness, oily skin, and pounding heartbeat. If the patient still had cold hands and feet or felt tired, I would add 50 mcg of T4 every two to three weeks, alternating between morning and afternoon doses until those remaining symptoms resolved.

More specifically, after the patient tried each dose for two to three weeks, I asked her to reassess her clinical status again. Perhaps on this second dose, she's now 25% improved. If she still had no adverse effects – but not complete resolution of symptoms – then the dose would increase again, increasing the noon dose by ½ grain (50 mcg) of T4. Once again, the patient would take this new dose and reassesses her clinical status after two to three weeks. Similarly, if there was an additional benefit and no harm, we continued upward in this gradual, step-by-step fashion until the optimal dose was found. Below is an example of the thyroid dose titration form filled out with the patient Jane Doe's goals in the column on the left and her initial dose titration schedule on the right. (Note: In this titration chart, "T4" refers to levothyroxine.)

Donna Hurlock, MD

Phone:555-555-5555

****Please notify me of any new problems****

Clinical Goals and Doses for JANE DOE **Date** JUNE 1

GOALS	BETTER	SAME
↑ ENERGY		
↑ WARM HANDS & FEET		
↓ WEIGHT		
↓ ANXIETY		
↓ PUFFY ANKLES		
↑ FOCUS		
↓ JOINT PAINS		
↓ BLOOD PRESSURE		
MOIST EYES		
↑ LIBIDO		
EVENING PULSE < 85		
↓ BLOOD PRESSURE		
↓ HAIR LOSS		

AM DOSE	LUNCH DOSE	TAKE FOR
ARMOUR 30	T4 50	2 weeks
ARMOUR 60	T4 50	2 weeks
ARMOUR 60	T4 100	3 weeks
ARMOUR 60/T4 50	T4 100	3 weeks
ARMOUR 60/T4 50	T4 150	3 weeks

Please follow schedule as written. Do not alter it. Only go as high as you need to feel well. Do not exceed the dose that makes you well. Report any problems to us by fax or email with the title "Thyroid Status Report."

Followup visit due: 3 MONTHS

Everything Jane Doe needed to do was clearly listed here, along with her goals and directions for how to follow the dose titration schedule. I also included my phone number to encourage the patient to call if any problems arose. At the bottom was the reminder for Jane to return for her first follow-up visit. This form worked quite well to help guide most patients in their search for their most therapeutic dose, and the copies helped me at follow-up visits to remember what specific goals were set for Ms. Jane Doe. Once we found the dose that achieved all those listed goals and did no harm, we knew we'd found her perfect dose!

YOU'VE FOUND THE OPTIMAL DOSE. NOW WHAT?

It's very rewarding for both the patient and the physician to reach this point where we've found the dose that eliminates most or all of the patient's initial symptoms! Whoo hoo! Better living through hormones!! If we're lucky, that dose will remain fully therapeutic for a long time. But, like many things in medicine and life, things change over time. Down the road, most patients will develop new symptoms suggesting underdose – and occasionally overdose – so the dose will need to be adjusted from time to time. That's why it's crucial NEVER to let down our guard. As I said before, patients and physicians need to continue paying attention to new developments and watch for signs of excess thyroid hormone. I can't emphasize enough how important it is to keep this in mind and for patients to communicate any new symptoms immediately so that the dose can be adjusted as needed. No matter how long it's been, the thyroid hormone dosage is *always* a work in progress!

CHAPTER 16: POTENTIAL HARM FROM EXCESS THYROID

"Everything in excess is opposed to nature."
~ Hippocrates

Patients taking too much thyroid hormone will become temporarily hyperthyroid. The extent of the effects and the potential for harm depends mainly on how long the situation continues. In this chapter, let's look at the potential risks and health implications of excess thyroid.

SIGNS AND SYMPTOMS OF EXCESS THYROID

Essentially, any symptom or clinical sign of hyperthyroidism can occur if the patient takes too much thyroid. Some of those symptoms are:

- Fast pulse or tachycardia
- Pounding heartbeat, chest tightness
- Heart arrhythmia
- Heart failure or heart attack (if the excess is very severe and very prolonged)
- Shortness of breath
- Puffiness
- Fatigue

- Heat intolerance
- Disrupted sleep and insomnia
- Tremor, hyperreflexia
- Jitteriness, anxiety, and irritability
- Restless legs, muscle twitching or tightness
- Diarrhea and loose stools, occasionally constipation
- Heartburn
- A voracious appetite or thirst
- Weight loss or weight gain
- Hair loss
- Oily skin, acne
- Bone loss
- Abnormally low cholesterol
- Mania and hypersexuality

I read somewhere that exophthalmos (bulging eyes) and other eye-related hyperthyroid symptoms were the exceptions to that rule. Still, I did have a patient who developed pain in one eye (without exophthalmos) that both her ophthalmologist and I suspected was thyroid related. When I stopped her thyroid medication, the symptom quickly resolved. That's the beauty of thyroid hormone; it's very short-acting, so any excess effect is easy to fix, particularly when we act promptly.

Whenever one of my patients developed new symptoms that could be due to her thyroid dose, to play it safe, I always assumed that her thyroid medication was the cause of the new symptom and stopped the treatment. If the new symptom was unrelated, stopping the dose had no effect (except for making the patient hypothyroid again.)

It was clear that a symptom was due to the thyroid dose when it quickly and fully resolved after discontinuing the thyroid medication. We would then resume our titration process, starting with a somewhat smaller dose, knowing that our optimal dose would be smaller than the dose that caused the problem.

USUAL TISSUE TARGETS OF T3 AND T4

I was taught in medical school that T3 is the "active" form of the hormone and that T4 is just the precursor hormone that needs to be converted to T3 to become "active." But in practice, they have different effects. After years of observing patients on thyroid replacement, I found that the symptoms of an excess of T3 or T4 hormone, while falling under the umbrella of hyperthyroidism, are often quite different. I believe that difference is partly due to receptors in specific tissues having different affinities for these hormones. Basically, some tissues may never lose their ability to convert T4 to the "active" T3, and others lose that ability.

T3 tends to stimulate the skin, hair, nails, conjunctiva, nerves, muscles, and the gastrointestinal tract. Some common symptoms of T3 deficiency include dry skin, itchy skin, dry, brittle hair and nails, dry eyes, sluggish reflexes, sluggish cognition, poor muscle tone, poor appetite, early satiety, heartburn, bloating, and constipation.

Some of the symptoms I noticed with excess T3 are neurologic symptoms like tremors, irritability, jitteriness, "hyperness," restless legs, eyelid twitch, etc. On exam, I often saw a tremor and hyperactive reflexes when testing reflexes. Excess amounts of T3 can also overstimulate smooth and voluntary muscle tissue, which can cause tight muscles, particularly around the neck and shoulders, tightness and spasms in the legs, and also spasms in the GI tract, which can cause swallowing difficulties, and sometimes constipation. Too much T3 can also overstimulate the GI tract, causing such things as an increased – sometimes voracious – appetite and diarrhea. So yes, too much T3 can cause both constipation and diarrhea. Sometimes the patient experienced bronchial tightening, which can cause shortness of breath, mainly associated with exercise. Some patients with excess T3 had heart contractions that pounded, even with a normal pulse. Irregularity of the pulse can be caused by both excess T3 and T4, but I usually suspected T3 in those cases. Hair is very sensitive to T3, and too much and too little both cause hair loss. Finally, since T3 tends to have a strong effect on the epithelium, it can sometimes cause oily skin, excessively soft and fine skin, acne, etc.

On the other hand, T4 tends to stimulate things we commonly tend to think of directly related to our metabolic rate. T4 deficiency makes you sluggish like your engine is simply not running. Symptoms that I usually linked to a deficiency of T4 were weight gain, fatigue, achiness, low temperature, cold intolerance, cold extremities, Raynaud's syndrome, slow pulse, slow cognition, disrupted sleep, etc.

I noticed that the symptoms of excess T4 were often related to pulse, body temperature, and sleep. For example, too much T4 is more likely to cause the patient's heart to race with an elevated pulse but without pounding. Also, too much T4 is more likely to make a patient feel hot and sometimes "hyper." In extreme cases, patients on too much T4 may look like they are on some stimulant drug. In addition, since T4 tends to be longer acting than T3, the midday dose of T4 is also more likely to make it harder to fall asleep. And sleep is almost always disrupted if the full afternoon dose is taken too late in the afternoon or the evening. Of course, if the dose of T4 is too high – or too high for too long – symptoms of excess listed above could eventually be seen.

The ability to differentiate between the effects of too much T3 and too much T4 helped me find the optimal dose of T3 and T4 for patients. For example, if my patient had some symptoms of T4 underdose – she was still cold, tired, and gaining weight – but at the same time had a symptom of excess T3 like a tremor, I significantly reduced the T3 (the likely cause of the tremor). After the hyperthyroid symptoms were gone, I'd increase the T4 a bit to make the patient warmer and more energetic without causing the tremor.

When initially deciding on what product to use for each patient, if predominantly T3 type symptoms were present, I tended to give some natural desiccated thyroid as a source of T3 to my patient, often mixed with additional T4. In contrast, if the patient was mainly just cold and tired, I tended to prescribe just T4. I also gave plain T3 and T4 to some patients, but as discussed earlier, synthetic T3 is very potent and "sharp" in its effect, giving a "burst" of stimulation that is sometimes too intense and short-acting. Natural desiccated thyroid seems to be a bit softer and smoother in its T3 effect. That's why I usually prefer natural desiccated thyroid as a source of T3 versus synthetic T3 (Cytomel). But because natural desiccated thyroid has a higher T3 to T4 ratio than one finds in a human, I found it necessary to "water down" the natural desiccated thyroid with some straight T4 to make the T3 to T4 ratio closer to that of a human.

Of course, as you might expect, some patients' bodies have not read these last few paragraphs. Specifically, sometimes patients get symptoms that can be interpreted as evidence of too much T3, but the patient is only taking T4, and vice versa. Therefore, it's crucial to be constantly observant and open-minded and never assume that these trends are universally true. These differences between T3 and T4 aren't set in stone. I did my best to keep an open mind and not fall into the dogma trap, remembering that each patient was different and didn't always respond the way I thought they would or should.

RISKS OF SHORT-TERM EXCESS DOSING ARE MINIMAL

What can happen if a patient is on too much thyroid for a short time? Interestingly, numerous reports from the 1970s and 1980s show how hard it is to cause serious damage with a one-time or short-term overdose of thyroid. Here are a few of their titles:

- "Benign course after massive levothyroxine ingestion," by Tenenbein et al. in 1986.[152]
- "Massive levothyroxine overdosage: high anxiety – low toxicity" by Gorman et al. in 1988.[153]
- "Minor signs and symptoms of toxicity in a young woman in spite of massive thyroxine ingestion" by Nystrom et al. in 1980.[154]

- "Acute thyroxine overdosage: two cases of parasuicide" by Matthews in 1993.[155]

In one 1977 report, "Thyrotoxicosis after a single ingestion of levothyroxine" by Hofe et al.,[156] a 31-year-old woman ingested 10 mg (10000 mcg) of T4 (about 100 times the current "standard" dose). She vomited but otherwise had a relatively benign course. None of these patients died, even though some were attempting to do just that. Fortunately, they picked the wrong drug to use for that purpose!

Finally, a 2015 Danish review of Poison Information Centre records[157] of patients who took up to 9000 mcg of T4 found that

> *"153 of 181 (85%) patients did not have symptoms of poisoning at the time of enquiry…there were no reports of long-term sequelae. Acute LT poisoning often follows a benign course….all symptoms resolved spontaneously without need of medical care."*

These reports illustrate that a short-term thyroid overdose is unlikely to cause any serious, long-term, or permanent adverse effects. This finding is quite reassuring. Still, we need to be alert to any symptoms of hyperthyroidism so that a woman isn't exposed to an excessive dose for a prolonged period of time, which can cause adverse effects.

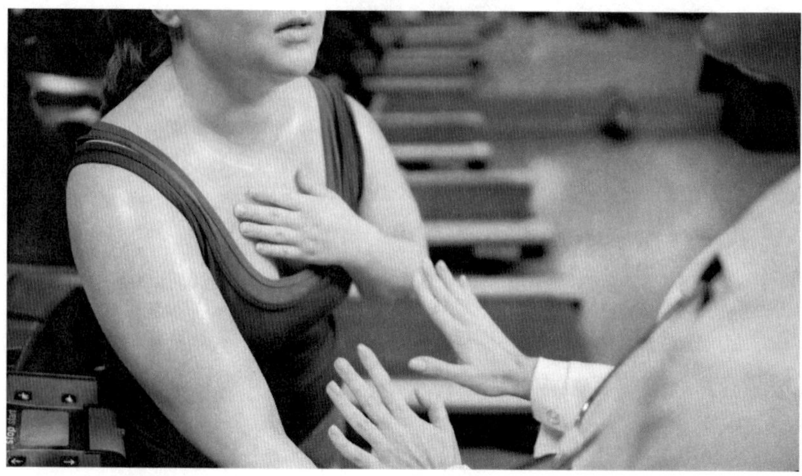

Again, I recommend that physicians make it clear to patients that they need to not only familiarize themselves with the signs and symptoms of overmedication but also agree to reach out immediately if they experience any symptoms suggestive of overdose. I also recommend that physicians document this warning very carefully in the patient's chart each time the warning is repeated for medicolegal reasons. I always fully documented these discussions. In addition, at the first visit, every new patient was asked to sign a specific "Thyroid Management Consent Form" that explained the risks in general terms. I found that signing the consent form also impressed upon patients the importance of self-monitoring for adverse effects.

I discussed diabetes treatment earlier in the book, but I'd like to call attention to how endocrinologists treat the two conditions differently. Some endocrinologists behave as if a mortal crime has been committed if a thyroid patient shows transient symptoms of thyroid overdose. They can even become quite belligerent when they see another physician tolerating a suppressed TSH! Yet, these same endocrinologists are nonchalant about the occasional insulin overdose, even though patients can go into hypoglycemic shock, require emergency care, and even die from an insulin overdose. In these doctors' minds, insulin overdose is an acceptable risk when managing a person with diabetes. But if they see a thyroid patient visit an ER with a suppressed TSH and transient heart palpitations that spontaneously convert to normal sinus rhythm within a couple of hours? OMG! It's *gross medical negligence!*

Why are they so emotional about too much thyroid – which is by far a safer hormone than insulin – and so accepting of insulin overdose, which is potentially fatal? Their divergent responses to these two situations simply make no sense! The answer is this: What they object to is that someone dares to disrespect their deity, the almighty TSH. Even though they have no data to show that TSH truly measures thyroid hormone function, it's like a religion to them. Thou shalt never suppress a TSH!!!

RISKS OF PROLONGED EXCESS DOSING CAN BE SIGNIFICANT

Most symptoms of overmedication, like jitteriness, heat intolerance, sleep disruption, etc., are mild, but they make patients uncomfortable. Consequently, they are quickly detected by the patient, who invariably reports those symptoms promptly to their physician. Temporarily stopping or reducing the dose always resolves these minor symptoms, so they are not reasons for significant concern.

But what happens when the symptoms aren't that noticeable or bothersome, and the patient takes too much thyroid hormone for an extended period? This is where real problems can occur. A longer period of thyroid hormone overdose will cause a condition analogous to naturally occurring hyperthyroidism, which is a situation you definitely want to avoid. The three most common categories of symptoms that potentially pose a significant risk to the patient are problems with the cardiovascular system, bone loss, and chronic diarrhea. We will discuss these below.

The first risk is to the heart. Specifically, excess thyroid hormone over time can trigger chest pain (angina), an abnormal heartbeat (atrial fibrillation) with the associated risk of blood clots, congestive heart failure, and in some cases debilitating or fatal heart attacks and strokes.

Years ago, I came across a case report from 1938 of an elderly gentleman with a history of a fragile heart who died of heart failure after being significantly overdosed with thyroid hormone for several weeks. During this time, he was experiencing daily chest pain, pounding pulse, shortness of breath, etc. Despite these symptoms, his physician did not reduce his dose. I can't locate that particular article so you can review it yourself. Still, it illustrates that severe adverse effects, including death, are possible with prolonged exposure to excessive thyroid hormone, especially in the case of an elderly gentleman with preexisting compromised heart function. The notable feature in this case was that despite the presence of fairly pronounced symptoms of overdose lasting for several weeks, those symptoms were *ignored.* Nothing was done to correct that excessive dose, which led to a fatal tragic – and likely very preventable – result.

To avoid cardiac toxicity, my approach was to have the patient monitor her pulse every evening, preferably with a method that will detect rhythm abnormalities. They were strongly and repeatedly reminded to promptly report the occurrence of any abnormal cardiac or other symptoms. They were also asked to report if the resting evening pulse began to average higher than around 85 beats per minute. That method was very effective at catching any problems early so we could change course and prevent big problems.

In preparation for writing this book, I searched the medical literature to find other examples similar to the one described above, where thyroid overdose led to a disastrous outcome for that older gentleman with preexisting heart disease. Reassuringly, my search revealed very few examples of severe complications. Most of the cases of thyroid overdose I found in the literature were of brief duration, and the symptoms resolved quickly after their dose was reduced or stopped. Happily, this suggests that severely bad outcomes are quite rare with over-replacement of thyroid hormone. Nevertheless, all adverse outcomes need to be avoided!

Another serious and adverse consequence of prolonged excess thyroid hormone is the development of osteoporosis.

If you remember the two ladies with severe osteoporosis we discussed earlier, you will have a clear idea of why it is vital to take great care not to cause bone loss by prescribing too much thyroid hormone. Since osteoporosis has no symptoms until something breaks, I regularly monitored my patients with bone density tests at the onset of thyroid replacement and every few years. If they began to show bone loss, we would screen the patient for all the possible risk factors that could cause the bone loss, starting with a re-evaluation of the patient's thyroid dose to ensure we aren't causing the bone loss with too much thyroid hormone. More often than not, either the patient had a low vitamin D level or wasn't on estrogen replacement, etc. Usually, the cause of the bone loss was not a thyroid dose that was too high. But it could be, so you should always consider that.

Finally, a less dangerous but quite debilitating consequence of taking excess thyroid over a prolonged period is chronic diarrhea, which we discussed earlier. It's sneaky because diarrhea often appears after a patient has been stable on her dose for a long time. I believe it's due to a gradual accumulation of T3 in the tissues, sensitization to T3, or improvement in T4 to T3 conversion. Nevertheless, it is easily remedied by simply stopping the thyroid dose. Then once the diarrhea is controlled and hypothyroid symptoms return, you can resume a smaller dose of usually just T4. But if the patient and her gastroenterologist do not notify you that it's happening, chronic diarrhea can be very disabling and can lead to weight loss, malnutrition, and any number of other significant consequences that we want to avoid.

This is why it's so important that patients are aware of the potential complications of excess dosage so that they can watch closely for the development of any signs that the dose is too high. In addition, physicians need to screen for the more dangerous results of overdose, such as heart rhythm and bone issues, by monitoring pulse daily and checking bone density every few years. In my practice, as soon as any problems developed, I was able to respond promptly by reducing or stopping the dose, thus allowing the hormone to wear off so that the symptoms of hyperthyroidism promptly disappeared. With physician vigilance and patient cooperation, severe complications should never occur.

WHAT TO DO WHEN AND IF THE DOSE IS TOO HIGH? STOP THE ENTIRE DOSE!

During dose titration, specific symptoms may suggest a patient is taking too much thyroid. These include heart palpitations, tremors, heat intolerance, disrupted sleep, a voracious appetite, and diarrhea. The absolute best way to eliminate those symptoms is to stop the entire dose immediately and let the symptoms resolve. I always reassured patients in this situation that their tissue thyroid level will not immediately plummet but will slowly begin to drop. I have never had a patient "crash" by doing this, and usually, the symptoms were gone within a few days, particularly if the patient had reported her symptoms to me promptly. While waiting for the symptoms to resolve, I also had a patient monitor her pulse daily and asked her to let me know as soon as her hyperthyroid symptoms were gone or if any new symptoms of underdosing appeared.

If she only needed a few days for the symptoms of excess thyroid to disappear, that indicated that she was on too much thyroid for a short time. When she resumed thyroid hormone, I'd recommend a dose around 25% lower than the previous dose. Also, if the symptom of excess were diarrhea or tremor – suggesting too much T3 – I also frequently eliminated T3 from her treatment. On the other hand, if it took weeks for the hyperthyroidism symptoms to wear off, she was likely on too much for at least a few weeks. So, after all the symptoms of overmedication were gone, I resumed with a significantly lower dose, frequently around half of the previous dose.

I was cautious not to resume thyroid treatment too soon or resume with a dose that was too high. Both of those errors would cause the hyperthyroid symptoms to quickly recur – something we wanted to avoid. When in doubt, my philosophy is always to start low and go slow. In the rare event that the apparent overmedication symptoms don't resolve, that was a sign that I needed to explore whether something else was going on that might be unrelated to a patient's thyroid status. Once we figured out what was going on and fixed the issue, the patient could resume her titration process while remaining *very* alert to any possible recurrence of those symptoms. Above all, symptoms that cause the patient to appear hyper should *never* be tolerated.

CHAPTER 17: ADDITIONAL THYROID DOSING CAUTIONS

"Medicine is a science of uncertainty and an art of probability."
~ Sir William Osler

I've shared a great deal of information on the hows and whys of my approach to dosing thyroid hormone. But I would be remiss if I didn't share a few additional cautions that physicians and patients should keep in mind when prescribing or taking thyroid hormone.

YOU MUST CONSTANTLY WATCH FOR SIGNS OF OVERDOSE!

Why am I emphasizing the importance of continued monitoring for signs and symptoms of thyroid overmedication, even after finding an optimal dose? There are several reasons:

- Patients' needs can change over time. For example, the absorption of thyroid medication can vary significantly in response to changes in dietary fiber intake or the new addition of medications and supplements, like antacids, ulcer drugs, or iron supplements.
- Thyroid hormone, particularly T3, can sometimes accumulate and saturate the tissues, causing overdose symptoms, even after a patient has been stable on a given dose for months or even years.

- The need for thyroid replacement can sometimes vary with the seasons and sometimes with alterations in sunlight and altitude.

It also appears that light exposure or Vitamin D, a hormone itself, affects our bodies' activation of thyroid hormone. Therefore, it's not surprising that if someone is suddenly exposed to a lot more sunlight than they are typically exposed to, like when they go to Florida for a vacation in the middle of winter, they are more likely to develop overdose symptoms. This happened to me when I lived up north and took winter beach vacations. And to maintain my current metabolic rate, I had to reduce my dose after I moved south to live in Florida. I always advised my patients to carefully watch for signs of overdose when they go to a sunny climate in the winter.

Similarly, I have had a few patients who seem to need less thyroid when they go to visit or live in higher altitude locations like Colorado. Perhaps that is also mediated through changes in sun exposure. I don't know why; I just know that patients should not stop monitoring their pulse and other possible signs of overmedication when they are away on vacation. In addition, quite a few patients seem to need more thyroid during the winter months, when the days are shorter. This is quite common, perhaps again related to fluctuations in Vitamin D and sunlight.

And finally, it's been my experience that some patients, particularly the ones who take just natural desiccated thyroid by itself, occasionally develop diarrhea after a few years. We discussed this earlier when we discussed thyroid's effects on the GI tract. They don't seem to have other overdose symptoms, but they do have unexplained diarrhea. More often than not, because the patient may have been stable for years on their current dose, it does not occur to them that their new problem with diarrhea could be due to their thyroid dose. When their gastroenterologist sends me a report about their diarrhea workup, I call the patient and advise them to stop their thyroid dose. Their diarrhea usually resolves within several days.

THE RISKS OF FINE-TUNING

When prescribing thyroid hormone replacement, there is always the possibility that a dose will be too high. This is a concern from both the clinical and medicolegal perspectives. Doctors don't want to ever do harm to our patients. However, this risk is a necessary evil when the goal is to find the optimal dose, especially when that dose is likely to be just slightly less than what would constitute an excessive dose. But I'll repeat it: as long as the patient and the physician pay attention and are willing partners in this process, actual harm is easy to avoid.

I like to compare finding the perfect dose to tuning a guitar. It's a trial-and-error process. If the string is too loose, the note will be flat, and if the string is too tight, the note will be sharp. Similarly, some trial-and-error adjusting is necessary to fine-tune the thyroid dose to get it perfect. Fortunately, thyroid hormone is generally relatively short-acting. If a patient has symptoms or signs of hyperthyroidism, it's easily and quickly resolved by lowering the dose to hit the perfect note. If we had a blood test that measured metabolic rate, we could use that to guide our doses. But until that is available, clinical response to each dose is our best guide.

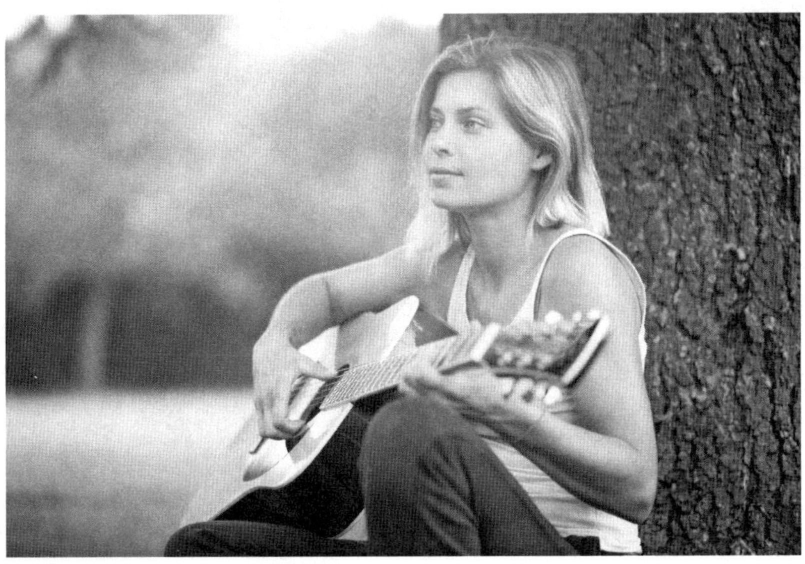

THE PATIENT MUST BE CONSCIENTIOUS AND CHECK HER PULSE DAILY!

To avoid harm from taking a dose of thyroid that is too high, patients need to understand that it's crucial to self-monitor their metabolism and promptly report any signs or symptoms of overdose to their physicians. The self-monitoring is essential because we don't want a patient to wait weeks or months for the next visit before the physician becomes aware of rapid pulse or other symptoms of hyperthyroidism. I can't live with a patient and check her pulse daily – but she can do it herself! I can't mount a camera to observe her for signs of hyperthyroidism throughout the day – but she can report them herself! My ability to carefully titrate the dose depends on the patient's observations and participation in this self-monitoring process. And to do that, she needs to know what symptoms to look for. As mentioned before, all my patients are given a printed list of common overdose symptoms at their first visit and are repeatedly reminded to watch for those things.

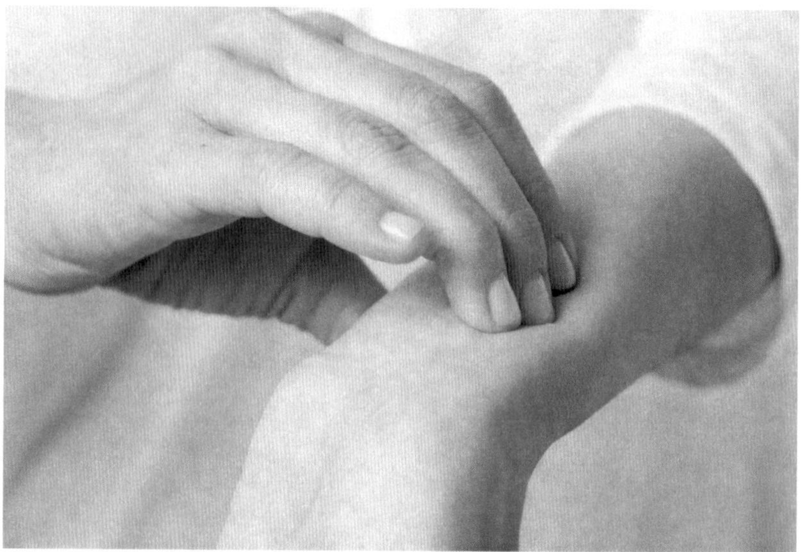

AVOID NON-COMPLIANT PATIENTS – KNOW YOUR LIMITS!

This is where it gets tricky. If the patient doesn't recognize her symptoms, isn't paying attention, or doesn't reach out to the physician, it puts everyone at risk. This problem is common among patients who lack the motivation to do their part in the process. Rather than monitoring and adjusting along the way, she overlooks and ignores symptoms until they become intolerable. Then, she's off to the emergency room. The result is an unhappy patient and a very offended and emotional endocrinologist or ER doctor…no fun.

My advice to patients: If you want to get well, you must be motivated and prepared to do your part. That means learning the signs and symptoms, daily self-monitoring, and swift communication with your physician.

And my advice to physicians: Don't attempt to fine-tune the thyroid dose with a patient who isn't highly motivated to get well or who is otherwise unable or unwilling to self-monitor. It simply puts you at too much risk. You should avoid patients who think they are the doctor, adjust their dose without consulting you, and only call when they run into trouble. Also, be cautious with hypothyroid teenagers. I found that as a group, they tended not to follow directions well. If they are not yet having serious problems from their hypothyroidism, I sometimes recommended that they wait a bit. With some maturity, I found that many of these young women eventually became more serious about their symptoms and were ready and willing to do their part in the thyroid dose titration process.

Patients with cognitive issues are also unlikely to succeed with thyroid dose titration unless they have a highly motivated and invested spouse, partner, or guardian who can do the monitoring for them. If a patient didn't have a support system and couldn't self-monitor, I didn't treat them. It was too risky for the patient and me. These patients are better off with a doctor who will manage them by blood tests. They will probably never become completely well using that approach, but at the same time, they aren't likely to ever become overdosed. And the physician won't have to deal with an angry endocrinologist, or worse yet, a lawyer bringing a lawsuit.

I went over the signs and symptoms list, line by line, with every new patient at their first visit and often repeated that process as needed. I also taught them to take their pulse with their fingers and note both rate and rhythm.

Keep in mind that taking the pulse should be done in the evening when a patient is at rest and the day's thyroid dose is still present and functioning. I always recommended it be done with the patient's own fingers, rather than devices like a Fit Bit or a blood pressure monitor, because those devices don't detect irregular beats. However, some handy state-of-the-art smartphone apps and devices like Kardia Mobile can get accurate information, including abnormalities in rhythm. The key is to use the same method daily, check the pulse daily, and report any problems promptly.

PATIENTS MUST REPORT PROBLEMS ASAP!

I told most patients that their average evening resting pulse should be less than 85. I did customize this somewhat, setting slightly lower cutoffs for patients on beta-blockers and slightly higher cutoffs for patients with a lifelong history of a higher pulse. If the pulse rate started to trend higher than their cutoff, the patient needed to call me immediately and stop taking their entire dose until we talked. The excess thyroid hormone needed to "flush out" of their system, which happens more quickly when they're not taking thyroid hormone than if they just lower their dose. The "flushing out" process usually takes only a few days. Once that is complete and the hyperthyroid symptoms are entirely gone, titration could continue, using a smaller dose than the one that caused the hyperthyroid symptoms. If the physician or patient is impatient and resumes thyroid hormone *before* the hyper symptoms are entirely resolved, symptoms will usually recur almost immediately.

In case I haven't emphasized it enough, *every* handout I gave to my thyroid patients always included the advice to CALL ME if any new problem appeared – even if the woman wasn't bothered by the symptom. For example, if the resting pulse was in the upper 80's, but they feel fine: CALL! Sadly, despite my multiple and repeated verbal and written warnings, some patients *still* didn't call! Instead, they'd try to manage it themselves, invariably by just lowering their dose a little rather than stopping their dose entirely. Because they were still taking most of the dose that caused the symptoms, and the excess hormone had not yet flushed out of their body, their hyperthyroid symptoms would often persist. They eventually let me know later, when they finally realized they had not fixed the problem. I would then remind them, again, that they need to contact me if at any point they feel that their dose needs to be reduced or if they simply have developed any new symptom. My friend Dr. Skinner had the same problem with his patients in the UK. He and I both agreed on the solution. If a patient repeatedly did this, we would discharge them from our practice to protect ourselves!

Patients who didn't tell me when they were having problems were the bane of my existence for years and put us all at risk. I wish I knew what exactly to say to those patients that would keep them from trying to deal with hyperthyroid symptoms themselves! I suppose I could have threatened them with refusing to take care of them, but that seems awfully harsh. Patients must be highly motivated, trustworthy, intelligent, willing to sign a consent form, and committed to self-monitoring and notification. Physicians should not attempt to use this dosing approach with patients who don't meet these criteria.

NEVER LET YOUR GUARD DOWN!

As in my prior analogy, if you tighten the string on the guitar much too tightly and keep tightening it, it will eventually break! Physicians and patients must always pay close attention and watch for signs and symptoms that suggest the dose is excessive. And if any symptoms of excess thyroid effect are discovered, act promptly by stopping the dose and letting the symptoms wear off.

Ultimately, here are my most important takeaways.

Patients: Your job is to pay attention to how your body is functioning, monitor your pulse every day forever for as long as you are taking any thyroid hormone, follow directions, and call your physician right away if you suspect that any symptoms of excess thyroid have developed. (And if you don't, and you continue to take an excessive dose of thyroid hormone for an extended timeframe, despite having symptoms of overdose, you could develop significant problems such as atrial fibrillation, etc., which could then lead to a clot forming in the heart, a stroke, or a heart attack!)

Physicians: Your job is to be smart, observant, and prudent, and to advise your patient to stop any excess dose until all those symptoms resolve, and then go low and go slow in the pursuit of optimal wellness – while *always* avoiding harm.

CHAPTER 18: THE TRUTH CAN CHANGE MINDS!

"In war, truth is the first casualty."
~ Aeschylus

Now that I am enjoying the freedom of retirement in beautiful Florida, I have the time to look back on the evolution of the practice of medicine since the 1970s, when I trained. I've concluded that, like many other aspects of our modern world, we are going in the wrong direction. In the war against underactive thyroid conditions, many physicians and patients are fighting what appears to be a losing battle! That's essentially why I wrote this book: To help change people's minds about what constitutes good hypothyroidism treatment and to better arm physicians and patients with the truth needed to fight the war against misinformation and poor treatment of hypothyroidism.

Over 100 years ago, when doctors first started treating hypothyroid patients with thyroid hormones, a careful clinical assessment was the standard – and only – way to assess a patient. Based on a patient's clinical history, physical signs and symptoms – and the physician's training and experience – an individualized treatment plan was made, and treatment was carried out. To determine if a treatment outcome was successful, you asked only one question: *Has the patient's health improved?*

There were no shortcuts, no surrogate markers, no batteries of random lab tests, no "physicals" where the patient is never actually touched by a doctor, no electronic medical records, no telemedicine, no "best practices," and no "expert clinical guidelines" to follow. Physicians received payment directly from a patient, and physicians' loyalty was, therefore, to patients. In essence, the patient *employed* the doctor. As a result, those physicians made every effort to do what was best for their employers: the patients! Physicians who were successful at making patients better were rewarded financially and usually had a full patient load. Meanwhile, those who failed to help patients saw their practices and incomes shrink. In my opinion, when the patient directly chooses and hires the physician, the resultant emphasis on patient outcomes and satisfaction is truly the best way to achieve quality control.

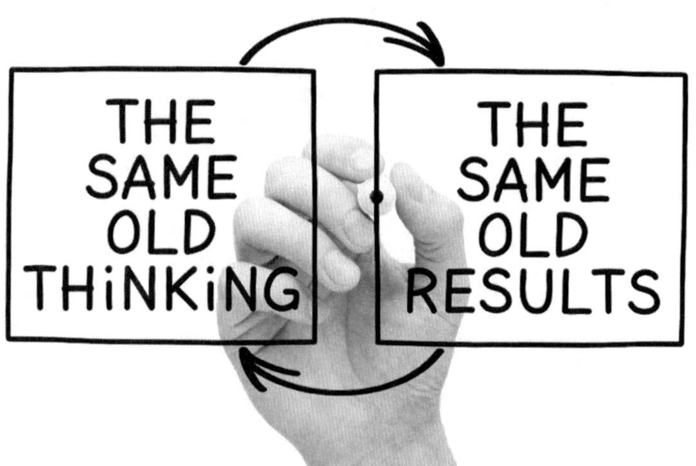

I was fortunate to have trained – and later practiced – under that first model. But today's physicians and patients aren't as lucky as I was. Currently, less than 30% of physicians own their own practices. Most physicians work for hospitals, HMOs, and other large medical corporations. By necessity, the loyalty of these doctors is to the businesses that employ them – *not* to their patients.

This new business of medicine puts physicians and patients in an undesirable and compromised position. For example, if a treatment is good for the patient – but *not* lucrative for the corporate employer – that treatment may never be recommended. Physicians are likely to be penalized by their corporate employers if they choose patients over profits.

Here's an example. A physician needs to send a patient for an MRI and knows that the best, most accurate, and state-of-the-art MRI machine is located several miles away. But the physician's corporate employer has a corporate-owned, in-house MRI facility, and it's known to be vastly inferior in quality. The physician will almost always *refer patients to the in-house facility because they'll be penalized if they don't.*

This is the primary problem with today's system of medical care. It's getting worse every year as state and federal governments, insurance companies, and large corporations exert increasing pressure on physicians to "comply" with their preferred practices. Many large groups even employ "compliance officers" to help herd their physician employees into recommended and required "best practices." Physicians are even encouraged to take continuing medical education (CME) courses that teach us how to best comply with a long list of onerous regulations. You can see that, as long as there are third-party payers for health care and physicians are "employed" and therefore regulated by these third parties, patient care will be compromised.

These corporations are run by bureaucrats and executives who often have little knowledge of medicine and little or no clinical skill or experience. As a result, these bureaucrats and executives have devised their own ways to evaluate "outcomes," with codes, programs, and "metrics" that quantify the "care" being provided by their employees. Those metrics rarely consider the individual patient's wellness, level of satisfaction, or the quality of the care they receive. Physicians who successfully treat or cure their patients don't get rewarded financially for their success under this model. Instead, they get to keep their jobs – or maybe even earn financial rewards – for rushing through a backbreaking daily quota of dozens of 7-minute patient appointments. They are also rated on their ability to control or even reduce costs, usually by avoiding additional diagnostic steps such as further testing or specialist consultations. Patient outcomes are rarely part of the equation.

For example, Medicare, as well as many health insurers and HMOs, will not approve and cover costs for any number of screening tests that may be helpful or even essential for a patient. If a physician orders a vitamin D level for a Medicare patient, a faceless and nameless Medicare bureaucrat can decide it's unnecessary. That physician can then be severely fined and punished by the federal government.

There's also a growing mob mentality among some doctors. If a "maverick" physician dares to treat patients in a manner that doesn't follow the current so-called best practices – *especially when the outcomes are superior for patients* – the mob feels threatened. They then mount coordinated campaigns to criticize and persecute other doctors. This has happened to some pioneering and beloved thyroid practitioners, such as my friend, the late Dr. Skinner, in the UK. Some of these doctors were mercilessly targeted not by their grateful patients but by local endocrinologists, reported to medical boards, and eventually forced out of practice.

The bottom line: To dare to treat an individual as an individual is no longer recommended or even tolerated in modern medicine. Deviation from the norm isn't accepted. Cookie cutter medicine is king.

Today's medical schools teach physicians to concern themselves with issues like "cost containment and global health" rather than how to evaluate a patient and figure out what is wrong with that person who is sitting across from them in their office. Meanwhile, "telemedicine" – which has a role – is increasingly considered the *only* way to provide health care for the masses. But how can a doctor evaluate skin texture, feel a pulse, or evaluate pitting edema via video or telephone? The simple answer is that they can't.

When the system of care prevents careful, hands-on clinical assessment, quality of care usually suffers. But as long as the outcomes focus on profits over patients and calculations over clinical outcomes, no one seems to care except the patients and the old-fashioned clinicians. The health care system increasingly ties their hands.

"Compliance with guidelines" creates another huge problem: medical innovation is entirely stifled. Many, if not most, medical advances over the years have occurred as a result of an individual physician trying something new that they suspect might help their patient, or perhaps the patient notices an unexpected benefit from a particular treatment. That benefit is reported as a case report, other physicians try the same approach and get good outcomes, and medical progress is made. When physicians are only allowed to follow their employers' best practices manuals and guideline requirements, no innovation can occur, and medical knowledge becomes stagnant.

This is exactly what has happened with thyroid management in the past several decades. Physicians are now expected to manage their thyroid patients solely by blood tests. Why? Because someone 50 years ago claimed – without any proof – that the TSH test is the best way to measure thyroid function. Corporate healthcare latched on to this idea partly because monitoring by lab tests alone is so much easier – not to mention time- and cost-saving – compared to taking the time needed to carefully evaluate patients and adjust their treatment as often as necessary to reach optimal relief of symptoms.

Instead of aiming for a patient's clinical wellness – as was done for at least half of the twentieth century – we are now required to use the surrogate marker, the TSH level, as our goalpost...*even if the patient is miserable*! And they *are* miserable! Survey after survey of actual patients with hypothyroidism, and post after post on social media, show that patients aren't happy with a TSH-based treatment approach.

My experience treating many thousand hypothyroid patients during my decades of practice is the same. Many women came to me after months or years of misery on ineffective thyroid treatment with other physicians. Their physicians' attention was not focused on resolving patients' symptoms but on normalizing the almighty TSH test. The clinical outcomes of patients didn't seem to matter much. This lack of concern seems to be particularly true among academic "experts." They seemingly worship their almighty TSH test and become incensed if anyone dares to question its validity or usefulness. Patients' feelings and long-term health outcomes aren't even part of the conversation.

It's a familiar pattern, actually. As I discussed earlier in the book, we saw the same thing happen with estrogen replacement in menopausal women. Back in the 1960s, when physicians encountered a newly menopausal woman who was miserable with hot flashes, vaginal dryness, and poor sleep, they offered full replacement of her gonadal hormones. This approach relieved the symptoms of deficiency, such as hot flashes, night sweats, and bone loss. And, as we later found, it also reduced heart disease and mortality. It was the standard of care and an excellent method to keep women healthy and happy. Further, reams of clinical data showed that women lived longer and felt better when their reproductive hormones were promptly and completely replaced.

But then, the powers that be – Big Pharma, along with certain government and academic physicians who were financially tied to Big Pharma – decided to upend that process by creating a massive trial called the Women's Health Initiative (WHI). The WHI was *designed* to make estrogen look bad. Why? Because estrogen was cheap and not very profitable, and they realized that HRT was too effective at preventing diseases like heart disease, osteoporosis, etc. That, in turn, was preventing sales of all those other wonderful and profitable drugs used to treat those chronic conditions.

So, in order to make estrogen look bad, they limited their patient population to older women with multiple risk factors for heart disease. And even worse, these women were, on average, 15 years *post* onset of menopause, a timeframe when women are *least* likely to benefit from estrogen replacement. Despite their best efforts at sabotage, the study *still* showed some benefit in the younger women in the trial, so the researchers then simply misrepresented those results and instead amplified the alleged risks. It's telling that the WHI trial received eight times more press than any other medical study that had ever been published.

The net result of this coordinated fear campaign aimed at menopausal women is that now, two decades later, most menopausal patients and their physicians still think HRT is dangerous. Rather than prescribing HRT to *prevent* conditions and symptoms related to an estrogen deficiency, physicians now prescribe a long list of other pharmaceutical drugs – medications for depression, anxiety, sleep problems, and osteoporosis – to *treat* conditions and symptoms *after* they develop.[158]

Similarly, without optimal thyroid hormone replacement, patients with hypothyroidism are more likely to develop a host of additional conditions and take multiple medications, including antidepressants, antianxiety drugs, statins for high cholesterol, sleep aids, diabetes drugs, and weight loss medications, among others.

The bottom line is that disease prevention has *never* been the ultimate goal of the pharmaceutical industry. Prevention is inherently bad for business. This is true for estrogen replacement in menopause and is equally valid for thyroid replacement in hypothyroidism. When both are done well, pharma profits are limited since patients no longer need dozens of drugs just to stay alive.

There is some good news, however. For now, physicians in this country still have the opportunity to provide their services directly to patients willing and able to pay directly for those services. For example, the Surgery Center of Oklahoma (https://surgerycenterok.com), a facility that accepts only direct payments from its patients, comes to mind. (Keep in mind that this isn't allowed in many countries with universal healthcare or socialized medicine, which is why many of their patients are

Canadians.) Even as medicine generally becomes more corporatized, an increasing number of physicians are opting out and using this model of practice. At the same time, more and more patients realize that it's the best and only way to restore genuine patient-centered quality health care.

Frankly, I'm increasingly convinced that to ensure that patients get the best care possible, we need to eliminate third-party payers for all out-patient care because they invariably interfere with the once-sacred doctor-patient relationship. So, for physicians, my advice is to "just say no" to big corporate conglomerates who want to employ you.

If you're a patient, remember that whoever pays the piper gets to choose the song. Similarly, whoever is paying for the healthcare gets to control the quality of that care. By avoiding the use of your insurance or HMO for your hypothyroidism care and seeking out physicians who are motivated and able to give excellent care – and whose actions aren't restricted by pressure from outside payers – *you* will finally get your hypothyroidism sufficiently treated and achieve the wellness you deserve.

Several groups such as The Wedge (www.jointhewedge.com), Gold Care (www.goldcare.com), and Thyroid Change (www.thyroidchange.org) either refer patients to such physicians or provide care from physicians who accept payments directly from their patients—and not from third-party payers.

By now, you know that I'm no fan of corporatized medicine. I do want to say, however, that on rare occasions, it can be done right. Paloma Health (www.palomahealth.com) is a virtual medical practice explicitly founded to provide high-quality, effective care *only* for hypothyroidism. Paloma's doctors serve patients in most states in the US, providing virtual visits, comprehensive home thyroid testing, and prescriptions by mail – as well as support for nutrition and lifestyle changes.

Paloma's doctors are highly knowledgeable about diagnosing and treating hypothyroidism, and the company's success – and the success of doctors in their practice – is based on *patient satisfaction!* (A novel concept, right?!) It can be a practical option, particularly for patients in areas of the country where thyroid-savvy physicians are in short supply.

IN TRIBUTE TO THE UK'S DR. GORDON SKINNER

I mentioned him earlier in this book, but before I finish, I wanted to take an opportunity to more fully honor the tremendous contributions of my friend and colleague, Gordon R B Skinner MD DSc FRCPath FRCOG. Dr. Skinner was a brilliant Scottish physician and researcher who changed *many* people's lives with his groundbreaking treatment of thyroid patients at his Birmingham, UK, clinic. Dr. Skinner and I approached hypothyroidism diagnosis and treatment in a very similar way. Sadly, his untimely death on November 26, 2013, left his many devoted patients throughout the UK without a doctor who would treat their thyroid disease correctly. Not surprisingly, the UK's rigid and dogmatic National Health Service doctors will only treat patients by lab tests alone. Those same doctors had regularly registered complaints about Dr. Skinner's methods (no doubt at least partly out of jealousy.)

My favorite passage from his book, *Diagnosis and Management of Hypothyroidism*, discusses the attitudes and practices of endocrinologists. When I read this passage, I still hear it in his classic Scottish brogue:

> *"I know this will make me unpopular with my Endocrinological colleagues but there seems to be an almost perverse pleasure in deeming that a patient isn't hypothyroid – usually on blood test results of which more anon – but also on a new principle that if other than an Endocrinologist considers a patient to be hypothyroid then that patient isn't hypothyroid even although my old Mum – who was not a medical practitioner but thought she was – would make the diagnosis."*

As I quoted Dr. Skinner earlier:

> *"It is staggering how many patients are patently hypothyroid but an Endocrinologist pronounces – often with some irritation – that the patient is definitely not hypothyroid and spouts cock about evidence-based medicine having omitted to take the patient's pulse or temperature or even listen to the woman."*

If you ever come across a copy of Dr. Skinner's fabulous book, I encourage you to buy it without hesitation. His charm, kindness, wisdom, and natural humor are on full display throughout his wonderful and insightful little blue book. I feel very fortunate to own several autographed copies of his book and to have shared one patient's care with him (an American who lived and worked in London.) I was also honored to be Dr. Skinner's guest in his home in Birmingham many years ago!

The world of hypothyroidism management lost a brilliant champion and a friend to many, as evidenced by this post from a writer in a thyroid support group:[159]

> *"He will be sadly missed by his family, friends, and thousands of thyroid patients whom he had helped to regain their lives through his diagnosis and treatment of hypothyroidism. Many patients became firm friends with Dr. Skinner, enjoying his quirky sense of humour and it is so sad that we will never be able to hear his lovely Scottish lilt again."*

Thyroid patients would be much better served if we had many more Dr. Skinners in this world!

A FINAL THANK YOU

Finally, I would like to thank you for taking the time to read this book. To my readers who are hypothyroid patients, I hope this book will help you understand the best way to manage your hypothyroidism and help you find a physician who can successfully help you get well…and who isn't afraid to do so.

And to my fellow physicians and healers reading this book, I encourage you to be brave but careful when you do what you know is in a patient's best interest. Fully inform your patients of the pros, cons, risks, and benefits, and document everything well. Do not tolerate patients who are careless with their dosing or try to adjust their dose independently. By doing those things, they are putting both themselves and you at risk. Insist that they inform you of any problems that might arise during their treatment. Above all, when it comes to assessing thyroid function in your patients, just like Osler said, listen to your patients because they will usually tell you what's wrong *if* they are just given a chance!

By now, you know that I love on-topic quotes, so I'd like to conclude with one from the famous playwright George Bernard Shaw:

> *"Progress is impossible without change; and those who can't change their minds can't change anything."*

Whether you're a patient or a physician, I hope this book has made inroads in helping you change your mind about the most effective way to diagnose and treat hypothyroidism.

True wellness is out there; it's up to us all to make it happen!

En bonne santé!

Donna G. Hurlock, MD
Venice, Florida

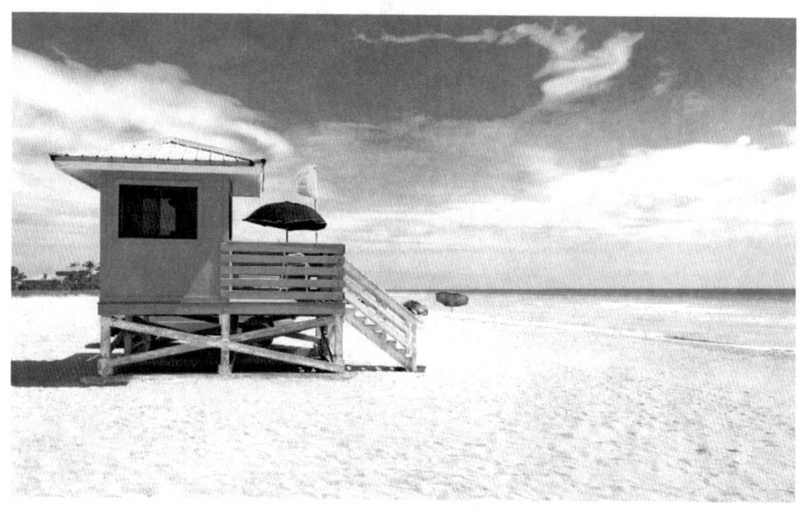

PART 4: APPENDIX

APPENDIX A: CLINICAL PEARLS OF THYROID WISDOM

After decades of successfully treating hypothyroid patients, there are some things I learned along the way I hope will be helpful to both patients and practitioners reading this book. This section summarizes some of my key recommendations regarding the successful management of hypothyroidism, listed in no particular order. (Remember, though, that we are all individuals, and these recommendations don't necessarily apply to *every* woman with hypothyroidism.)

DO THE MATH

You'll find many different equivalency charts showing conversion for levothyroxine (T4) drugs versus liothyronine (T3) and natural desiccated thyroid (NDT). After years in practice and trial and error with thousands of patients, I ended up deciding on the following equivalency/conversion:

1 "grain" of thyroid equals:

- 60 mg of NDT
- 100 mcg of T4
- 25 mcg of T3

Clearly, a cup of cashews is not exactly the same as a cup of peanuts or mixed nuts, but you get the idea.

GIVE IT TIME

Smaller doses of thyroid hormone replacement can be tried for as little as two weeks, but larger doses should be given a more extended trial time since the effect sometimes accumulates over time. In doses higher than 90 mg of NDT (1.5 grains) twice a day, I generally have the patient try each dose for at least three to four weeks before considering an increase.

MIX T4 AND T3

Using only natural desiccated thyroid or straight T3 may eventually lead to symptoms of T3 excess in many patients. I've found that most patients respond better to a mix of both natural desiccated thyroid (or a straight T3 drug like liothyronine/Cytomel) with *some* levothyroxine.

SPLIT DOSES EVENLY

Keeping the early morning dose and the lunchtime dose about equal in amount works well for most people. For example, 90 mg (1½ grains) of natural desiccated thyroid taken after waking works well with 150 mcg (1½ grains) of T4 taken with lunch in many patients.

DOSE TWICE A DAY FOR WEIGHT CONTROL

When controlling weight is an issue, I've found that taking two daily doses works much better than just a single dose in the morning. Twice-a-day dosing seems to help burn calories for more hours during the day and may also inhibit the hunger that often occurs in the mid-afternoon when a single morning dose is usually wearing off.

DON'T WORRY ABOUT DOSING WITH MEALS

Taking thyroid medication with meals isn't a significant problem if your goal is clinical wellness and relief of symptoms. It's only a problem if your goal is a perfect TSH level.

SEPARATE DOSES BY FOUR TO SIX HOURS

The first and second doses of the day should be taken about four to six hours apart.

DOSING TOO LATE WILL DISRUPT SLEEP

In general, each dose of thyroid medication provides about eight hours of energy. The second dose should be taken at lunchtime or earlier in the afternoon; taking the medication in the late afternoon or evening can disrupt sleep. (That said, some patients can tolerate a small late afternoon or evening dose or even find it helpful for sleeping.)

WATCH FOR 3 A.M. WAKING

If a patient has an easy time falling asleep but awakens at 3 a.m., this is a sign that more T4 is needed at lunchtime.

CONSIDER INCREASING THE DOSE DURING COLDER MONTHS

Some patients need a little more thyroid hormone during winter compared to summer months. (But patients taking extra thyroid during the winter should be aware that if they have a winter getaway to a hot, sunny climate, they should monitor themselves for symptoms of hyperthyroidism. As I mentioned, I suspect extra vitamin D from sun exposure potentiates thyroid function.)

SUPPLEMENT WITH VITAMIN D

Speaking of Vitamin D, studies show a reduction of antithyroglobulin antibodies and a reduction of TSH when vitamin D is given to study subjects who have Hashimoto's thyroiditis.[160] Clinically this translates into a simple fact: the thyroid function of some patients *improves* when the patient takes a vitamin D supplement regularly.

I've always encouraged all my patients to supplement with around 5,000 IU of vitamin D daily. A serum level of 50 ng/dl is a good goal for Vitamin D. (This is about the mid-point of the reference range at many labs.) If you want to learn more about vitamin D, I recommend reading *The Vitamin D Solution*, written in 2011 by Dr. Michael Holick.[161]

PAY ATTENTION TO HOW ESTROGEN TREATMENT AFFECTS THYROID

I hope that at this point in the book, I've made it clear that the presence or absence of estrogen can have a major effect on thyroid replacement.

The forms of estrogen most likely to affect thyroid hormone dosing are HRT pills and birth control pills. Oral estrogen increases the production of sex hormone binding globulin, which binds and inhibits thyroid hormone. While still possible, it's less likely with transdermal estrogen products like patches, creams, and implantable pellets.

That said, here are two guidelines to keep in mind.

Women on an optimal dose of thyroid medication who *start* supplemental estrogen or increase their dose of estrogen may find that their thyroid medication becomes less effective. Those women usually need a slight increase in their thyroid hormone dosage to regain their prior level of wellness and symptom relief. In general, women who are taking any form of estrogen will need a higher dose of thyroid hormone than women who aren't taking estrogen.

Women who are on an optimal dose of thyroid medication *and* supplemental estrogen and then *stop* taking the estrogen should watch closely for the development of any signs or symptoms of thyroid overdose. Their dosage of thyroid hormone may need to be reduced.

PAY ATTENTION TO HOW THYROID TREATMENT AFFECTS ESTROGEN

The presence or absence of thyroid hormone also affects estrogen therapy.

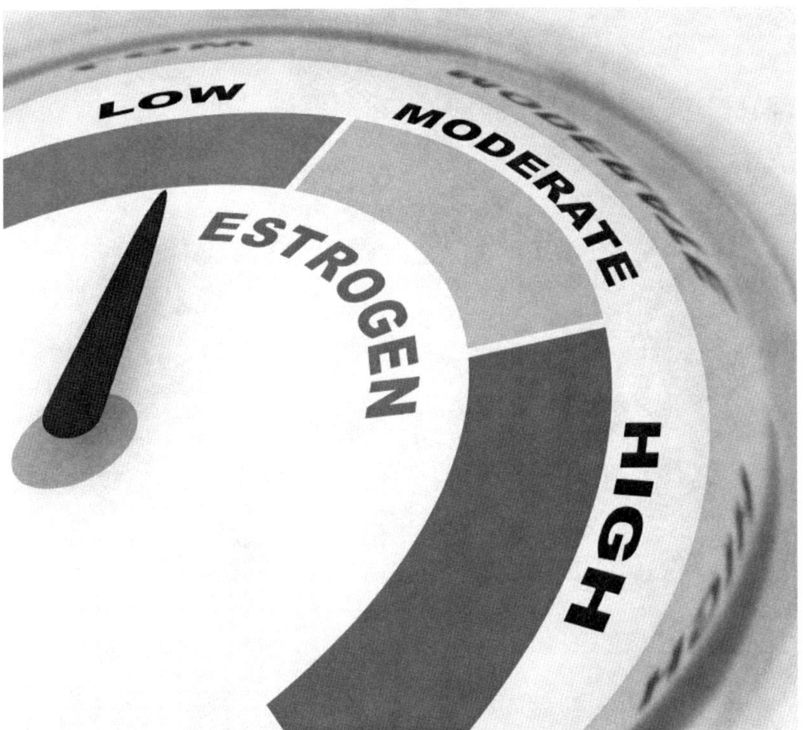

Women who are on a stable and optimal dose of supplemental estrogen and then start thyroid medication – or increase the dose of thyroid medication – may notice a change in the clearance of estrogen that makes the estrogen less effective. Because of this, as thyroid medication is introduced or the dosage increased, it's a good idea for those women to watch for the recurrence of menopausal and related estrogen deficiency symptoms. They may need an increase in the estrogen dosage.

Let's use an example of a woman who is feeling well and controlling hot flashes on ½ of a .1mg estradiol patch. She starts thyroid hormone replacement – or increases her dose of thyroid medication – and as she gets close to the optimal dose of thyroid medication, her hot flashes return. In this situation, I would usually increase those patients to a full .1 mg estradiol patch.

BE CAREFUL ABOUT ANTI-SEIZURE DRUGS AND BLOOD THINNERS

For patients on anti-seizure drugs or blood thinners – where the serum level needs to be maintained at a certain therapeutic level – there's a caution. Adding thyroid medication will usually *increase* the rate at which the body breaks down those other drugs, making them *less* potent. When thyroid replacement is newly prescribed in these patients, the doctors prescribing those other medications should be alerted, as they may need to increase the dosage of those drugs to maintain the same serum levels.

DON'T WEAN OFF OTHER MEDICATIONS UNTIL THYROID TREATMENT IS OPTIMAL

If a woman with hypothyroidism wants to get off of other medicines that have been prescribed to control various symptoms of hypothyroidism – for example, antidepressants, ADHD medications, statin drugs, or sleep aids – I always encouraged the patient to start that process only *after* the optimal dose of thyroid is identified. That way, we only change one thing at a time, making each dose's effects easier to assess.

DON'T START OR STOP SUPPLEMENTS WHEN TITRATING THE THYROID DOSE

I have the same advice for supplements. When a patient starts or stops one or more supplements simultaneously as they go through the thyroid titration process, it's extremely difficult to determine which product is responsible for any side effects. Therefore, it's always best for patients not to change anything else during thyroid titration. (The beauty of that is that often, once the optimal dose is discovered, many or most symptoms may disappear, and those supplements aren't even necessary anymore!)

CONSIDER A TRIAL OF THYROID HORMONE DURING CHEMOTHERAPY

Based on years of observation, I believe that chemotherapy often damages thyroid function. The job of chemotherapy is, after all, to kill cells that are reproducing. Because chemotherapy usually doesn't affect the TSH level, this cause-and-effect correlation is rarely acknowledged, much less diagnosed. I suspect that this may even be part of the mechanism by which cancer patients lose their hair and appetite and develop symptoms like "chemo brain" and prolonged fatigue...all symptoms of hypothyroidism as well.

Since modern medicine lacks good ways to control these side effects of chemotherapy, it would seem that a trial of thyroid might be helpful when you see these symptoms, even when the TSH level is normal. In support of this concept, I have noted that my well-replaced thyroid patients who later needed chemotherapy tended to tolerate their cancer treatment much better than other patients who aren't on thyroid. My well-replaced thyroid patients also had fewer side effects when taking chemotherapy drugs.

BE AWARE OF THE TSH/CHOLESTEROL LINK

Most hypothyroid patients who are on an optimal dose of thyroid will, in my experience, have a TSH value close to 0 and will often achieve cholesterol values of around 165 mg/dl. When the dose of thyroid medication is lowered to normalize the patient's TSH level

– something I regrettably did all too often early in my practice – the patient will lose significant clinical benefits they have achieved. Their cholesterol values will go back up into abnormal ranges. (A note for doctors: When a patient's hypothyroidism is resolved, and their cholesterol magically drops, their primary care physician will likely *not* thank a doctor like me for lowering the cholesterol levels of the hypothyroid patients because they rarely know that cholesterol and thyroid function are linked. They *will,* however, be upset when the TSH is suppressed!

FREE T3 LEVEL IS THE MOST HELPFUL OF THE LABS

Although I do not recommend using thyroid lab tests to determine the best dose of thyroid replacement, the one lab that seems to be at least somewhat correlated with thyroid function is Free T3. In my experience, patients are usually not well if the Free T3 level is less than 3.0 pg./ml, around the mid-point of the reference range.

There are exceptions to this rough generalization, however, so don't depend on it as a shortcut to determining the optimal thyroid dose. Ultimately, I always prefer that we measure thyroid function by assessing a patient's wellness via a thorough clinical evaluation. That's the best way to avoid overdosing or underdosing patients and optimize wellness for the long-term – the ultimate goal!

APPENDIX B: CLINICAL EXAMPLES OF THYROID DOSING

I'm sharing these clinical examples of how I managed some former patients to illustrate my approach to thyroid hormone replacement. I chose these patients because each woman had a particularly interesting clinical presentation or outcome. A few were quite complicated. Hopefully, this will tie together the concepts I've presented in this book and help patients and practitioners understand that while it can be a complex process, you can achieve effective hypothyroidism treatment with patience and perseverance. (Please note that I've used pseudonyms to protect patient privacy.)

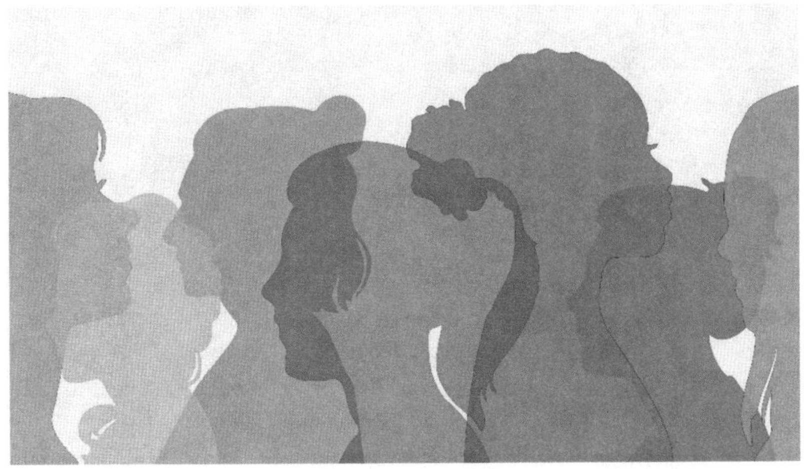

"ALEXANDRA"

One of my first thyroid patients was an instructional technologist, Alexandra, who had been a skinny professional ballerina during her teenage years. Due to her low weight, as is common in ballerinas, her periods had not begun until age 19, after she finally stopped dancing professionally and gained some weight. After she began having regular periods, she started taking birth control pills for contraception. She came to see me at age 26 for routine gynecologic care unrelated to her hormonal status. She was married, 5'6" and 142 pounds at that time, and still on the pill. Then at age 31, she decided she wanted a baby, and to prepare for that, she dropped her weight to about 130 pounds.

She discontinued her birth control pills, hoping to conceive, but she had no menstrual periods after stopping the pill. Her lab tests showed Prolactin of 9.1, TSH, 5.59, FSH 7.1, LH 7.5, and her Beta HCG was negative. Alexandra was referred to a reproductive endocrinologist. Despite Alexandra's TSH of 5.59 – a level many doctors would consider abnormal and therefore treatable – the endocrinologist ordered more lab tests and advised Alexandra to eat a high-protein, low-carb diet. The doctor also prescribed some estrogen for suspected hypothalamic amenorrhea. The plan was to give her a small dose of Synthroid for the "slightly elevated" TSH and some medication to induce ovulation. She was also scheduled for a complete infertility workup.

When I saw her in the office about three months later, Alexandra was still not having periods and had gained back all of those 12 pounds she had lost, despite a very small appetite. She had not yet been started on thyroid medication by her reproductive endocrinologist. Her weight was now back at 142 pounds, and she was tired. She also had very dry skin that was breaking out, significant hair loss, and yellow palms. (Beta carotene intake from eating carrots does not break down very fast in hypothyroid patients, which can cause the palms to be yellow.) It was clear to me that she needed thyroid replacement. Due to the prominence of the skin and hair symptoms and sluggish gut, I thought Alexandra would benefit from a thyroid dose that included a good amount of T3. So, after discussing the plan with the reproductive endocrinologist, I started her on 30 mg of Armour Thyroid once a day and then increased her to 60 mg once a day. (At that time, I did not yet appreciate the value of twice-a-day dosing.)

About 10 weeks later, Alexandra came in for a follow-up and reported that she was feeling better and having significantly less hair loss. She was now down to 136 pounds with a pulse of 74 and no symptoms of excess thyroid. Her TSH was now .061 with a low T4 and a high T3. Again, because I was still new at managing thyroid at this time, I still believed that these labs were necessary. So, despite an excellent clinical result, I switched her to 125 mcg of Synthroid daily in an attempt to normalize the labs. She was advised to watch for symptoms of overdose.

One week later, Alexandra called to report some spontaneous spotting. A sonogram showed a classic image of polycystic ovaries with a normal endometrium. Several weeks later, she said she was again losing hair and now was constipated. Later in my career, I would have resumed some T3 for those symptoms, but back then, my response was to increase the Synthroid dose slightly to 150 mcg daily. But then I made the mistake of doing another TSH, which was still low at .015, so I advised her to reduce her dose to 125 mcg of Synthroid daily.

Two months later, Alexandra had a spontaneous period! How exciting! TSH was still low at 0.022, and the plan was to reduce the dose again to 100 mcg of Synthroid daily (to normalize the TSH, despite a great clinical result!) But a month later, she complained of fatigue and cramps. However, we quickly discovered that the cramps were due to the small fetus growing happily inside her uterus!!! Looking back, we should have just stayed with Armour Thyroid 60 mg daily, and I regret that I reduced her dose slightly in an effort to normalize her TSH value because that could have harmed the pregnancy. Fortunately, it did not, and Alexandra delivered a healthy, 7-pound, 7-ounce baby girl later that year without any fertility treatments. All she needed was some thyroid hormone to stimulate her metabolism and break down her reproductive hormones, allowing her to ovulate on her own and conceive. In her thank you note to me for helping her conceive, Alexandra wrote, "The Synthroid 100 mcg did the trick." Indeed, it did!

This is how many women with infertility were successfully managed back in the 1950s. Lucky for them, they did not have thyroid labs to worry about and test results that would prevent their doctors from giving them enough thyroid to resolve their symptoms. Knowing what I know now, I think we were lucky to have gotten such a great result with this patient since her tiny dose was likely not optimal (too small and not enough T3.) But sometimes you get lucky!

"LAUREN"

Lauren was a 50-year-old engineer for a defense contractor who I first saw in 2001 to have her estrogen replacement regimen managed. She was 5' 7 7/8" tall (yes, that's what she wrote!), and her weight was 122 pounds. Although she was quite thin, she generally appeared healthy. Lauren had already seen multiple doctors, including neurologists, pulmonologists, osteopaths, and several internists, but wanted yet another opinion. She was already on "Triest 2" transdermal cream (a compounded bioidentical estrogen product), progesterone, B12 injections, and a fairly restrictive anti-fungal diet. She had also recently been given a provisional diagnosis of Lyme disease the prior year after a tick bite that left a red mark. Her symptoms included swollen lymph nodes under her arm, pain in her eye, tingling in the scalp and toes, stiff joints, and numbness in her right leg. Lauren also woke up with a vibrating sensation throughout her body every two hours. Antibiotic treatment had not helped.

Further history revealed that her periods had ceased the previous August, and she occasionally had hot flashes. The Triest cream had helped her symptoms by about 50%. She also felt malaise and was sometimes tearful. Her TSH at that time was 2.0.

Around that time, the Women's Health Initiative Writers Group was slandering traditional HRT and sowing terror in the hearts of menopausal women worldwide. The result was a widespread fear of pharmaceutical HRT products. Compounded transdermal estrogen products were becoming very fashionable. They were marketed as somehow safer than pharmaceutical HRT products, even though no data showed that those products were safe or even effective. Another "benefit" being touted was that they rarely caused symptoms like vaginal bleeding. This "benefit" was, in reality, a sign that the doses being prescribed, particularly by non-gynecologists, were incredibly small. So yes, they did not cause bleeding, but these tiny doses also failed to adequately treat symptoms of menopause.

My initial approach was to replace the Triest cream and progesterone with a combo HRT product called Activella that contains a smallish (but not tiny) dose of estradiol and a normal amount of progesterone. Because Lauren's breasts became very sensitive to the small dose of estrogen and progesterone, we cut that pill in half, and I began to suspect that her thyroid function was deficient because most women would not develop breast soreness on such a small dose of estrogen.

Further questioning revealed that Lauren had significant fatigue, foggy memory, depression, mood swings, occasional palpitations, nausea for no reason, burning feet, and unrefreshing sleep. In addition, her basal body temperature was a bit low. Therefore, I advised her to do a trial of thyroid replacement. Lauren was an avid reader of all things alternative, so before considering that approach, she sought several more opinions and first tried various other non-pharmaceutical options to treat her symptoms.

When she came in for a pap smear in 2002, her hands and feet were cold, and her pulse was 56. She took a miniscule dose of her Activella (1/4 of a pill every other day) and still had many of her initial symptoms—though her sleep was somewhat improved. Once again, I advised a trial of thyroid, and we started with only 15 mg (1/4 grain) of Armour Thyroid once a day. Lauren had moderate improvement with that small dose but was reluctant to try an increased dose. Five years later, she stopped her HRT and her thyroid at the advice of a nurse friend. Lauren returned to my office, feeling worse. She was tearful, panicky, and foggy-brained, and her hot flashes had returned. Her hands and feet remained cold, her pulse was 60, and she weighed 118 pounds. I encouraged her to resume her prior regimen, which she did. She also started Wellbutrin for her depression but eventually, after she was brave enough to increase her thyroid dose to 15 mg twice a day, she was able to get off the Wellbutrin.

By 2011, due to fear of estrogen supposedly causing breast cancer – a reminder: it doesn't! – and due to her husband and best friend, the nurse, encouraging her to stop her HRT, Lauren was now back to the Armour Thyroid 15 mg dose once a day and was only using a tiny dose of compounded estradiol vaginal cream. In addition, she was now taking Vitamin D, C, and B12, quercetin chalcone, turmeric, B12, Bone Guardian calcium, Oncoplex (sulforaphane glucosinolate), "Brain Support" Ginkgo Biloba, phosphatidyl serine, acetyl L carnitine, DHA, choline, inositol and Kyodophyllus 9.

Sadly, despite my repeated attempts to increase her hormone doses, Lauren continued on this regimen of inadequate thyroid and inadequate HRT and continued for years to have significant vaginal discomfort. She blamed her vaginal issues on an alleged yeast infection, most likely due to vaginal atrophy due to inadequate estrogen replacement. She also developed osteoporosis due to estrogen deficiency and perhaps due to nutritional factors. In addition, her mood and energy remained low, anxiety high, constipation, and some neuropathy symptoms persisted, and her cholesterol remained above 200. As one might expect, Lauren's TSH remained normal at around 2 throughout this time.

Clearly, this isn't a very satisfying example of proper thyroid management. Lauren never achieved total wellness, primarily due to her intense fear of hormones and criticism from friends and family. As a result, she never allowed herself to do a proper trial of thyroid and continued to shy away from doses of HRT that would have helped her vagina, bones, and brain to stay healthy. Despite over a decade of her sincere attempts to achieve wellness plus my best attempts to counsel and educate her and guide her to wellness,

I could never get Lauren past her deep-seated fear. That fear prevented her from taking doses that would have helped her, thus perpetuating her lack of wellness. It's a shame, but it does teach us that we can't always cure everyone, no matter how hard we try.

"DORIS"

Doris was a labor nurse I had worked with when delivering babies early in my career. She first came to my office at age 42, after taking three months of Premarin .625 mg daily, prescribed by another physician. The other physician diagnosed her with early menopause, despite her normal FSH of 5.9. (This suggests that estrogen was not deficient.) She had previously had a hysterectomy, so she had no periods. Doris's primary symptoms at this time were occasional hot flashes, dryness of the vagina, and "all over" dryness, cold intolerance, cold hands, and thinning hair. She was also having some shortness of breath from time to time and some pain with sex. She had elevated cholesterol of 228 despite a weight of 120 pounds, a good diet, and a history of chronic benign hyperbilirubinemia – elevated bilirubin without an obvious cause and adverse effects. She appeared healthy other than signs of a vaginal yeast infection. Her pulse was 62 and regular, her blood pressure was 118/73, her height was 5'5". and her TSH was previously normal, at .874.

At that time, I was not sure if Doris was menopausal or not, but I did suspect she was hypothyroid and clearly had a vaginal yeast infection that needed to be treated. I planned to treat the yeast and increase the estrogen dose to .9 mg in case she was indeed menopausal, and the current dose of .625 mg was not enough for this young, thin woman. We also started a trial of Armour Thyroid. We repeated her TSH; this time, it was 3.341 with a free T3 of 2.89. Both of those values are "normal," but I considered both to be very suspicious.

Doris had some improvement in energy on 60 mg (1 grain) of Armour Thyroid daily but had some chest discomfort and an increase in the frequency of headaches on 90 mg (1½ grains) of Armour Thyroid, so she discontinued it not long after starting it.

But because her low thyroid symptoms persisted, she decided to try it again and stayed on a dose of 30 mg (½ grain) of Armour Thyroid twice a day. We also increased the Premarin dose to 1.25 mg because I suspected that Diane's chest discomfort and increased headaches could have been due to the thyroid hormone metabolizing away the small dose of estrogen she was taking. That increase in estrogen dose seemed to have worked. Her energy was improved, she was not nearly as cold, and with the increased estrogen, she no longer had any chest discomfort or significant headaches. Excellent!

Doris stayed on this dose for several years but later had some palpitations, which initially seemed to have worsened when she stopped her thyroid dose. Her shortness of breath also returned when she stopped her thyroid. Cardiac evaluation diagnosed mitral valve prolapse (MVP) with mild mitral regurgitation and normal sinus rhythm with rare premature ventricular beats. Cardiac evaluations failed to reveal any significant pathology. Doris decided to stay off thyroid due to fear of those MVP palpitations. Fortunately, she continued her full-dose estrogen replacement. Consequently, with that, plus an excellent diet and lifestyle, Doris maintained generally good health without thyroid replacement. However, her cholesterol remained high, and she continued to have cold hands and feet, which she simply tolerated.

"JENNA"

Jenna was discussed earlier during our discussion of thyroid hormone's effect on appetite and digestion. Jenna's mom brought her to see me for a thyroid evaluation when Jenna was 11. Her mom was a drug representative who called on me and was familiar with my practice and approach. Jenna's primary problem was delayed emptying of the stomach and chronic constipation. A pediatric gastroenterologist had done a full workup, including several colonoscopies and endoscopies, and diagnosed her with gastroparesis. The treatment was Pepcid, which Jenna took occasionally.

Jenna's other symptoms included chronic ear infections, a past case of pneumonia, many drug allergies, chronic and severe cold intolerance, fatigue requiring excessive amounts of sleep, dry, itchy skin, and some hair loss. She had ear tubes inserted at 6 months and permanent ones placed at age 2. She was petite and thin and weighed 64 pounds at a height of 4'8.5". Her temperature was 96.2, her pulse was 88 and regular, and her blood pressure was 99/70. Her hands were icy, and she appeared very tired during her visit, even resting her head on my desk. Her TSH was perfectly normal at 1.069.

Due to the dominant symptom of sluggish bowel function, I started Jenna on a trial of Armour Thyroid. Also, because her lifelong history of gastrointestinal problems would likely cause long-term nutritional deficiencies, I sent her for a bone density test. Her bone density showed that her spine was 21%, and her hips were 15%, less dense than normal for her age. After several dose adjustments, we found that a daily dose of 75 mcg of Levoxyl significantly improved her digestion and energy levels.

However, to further improve digestion and address residual hair loss, I increased Jenna's Levoxyl dose to 88 mcg per day and added 2.5 mcg of Cytomel. She continued to improve. At age 13, to simplify her dose, Jenna was changed to 50 mcg of Levoxyl twice a day, and this was later increased to ½ of a 125 mcg Levoxyl pill twice a day. By age 14, she was well on just ½ of a 137-mcg tablet of Levoxyl twice a day. TSH on this dose was barely suppressed at 0.184. Later we increased her dose to 75 mcg twice a day. To further stimulate peristalsis, we had tried several times to add a small amount of Cytomel or Armour Thyroid over the years. But, at this dose range, she repeatedly responded with an elevated pulse to both Cytomel and Armour, so we returned to just Levoxyl.

Happily, with thyroid therapy, Jenna could eat normal amounts of food, even requesting a snack after school. Her follow-up bone density done approximately 16 months after her first scan showed 14% growth in her total hip density and 21.4% in the spine! She also grew 4' taller and gained 26 pounds during that time! In addition, as evidence of good nutritional and hormonal status, Jenna's periods started at a normal age!

It was very disheartening that gastroenterologists had put young Jenna through all those invasive GI tests only to reward her with a diagnosis – *but no real cure.* Instead, if they had only listened to her symptoms and ignored her misleading TSH test, they could have avoided all those awful procedures and easily cured her GI symptoms with the small amount of thyroid I prescribed! It's a shame what's happened to our clinical skills since the introduction of these thyroid blood tests.

"AUDREY"

Audrey, a realtor, first came to see me at age 34, requesting a thyroid evaluation. Her father, a psychologist, suspected low thyroid function. Her symptoms included irregular and heavy periods – previously diagnosed as "polycystic ovarian syndrome (PCOS) – and chronic fatigue, achiness, puffiness, cold intolerance, constipation, poor sleep, and depressed moods. She also had a diagnosis of ADHD. Audrey was too tired to work at a normal pace. Her blood pressure was 115/78, her pulse 72, and she weighed 179 pounds at a height of 5' 10.5". She generally appeared healthy but had very cold hands. Her initial TSH was normal at 1.274, and her cholesterol was 228.

I started her on a trial of Levoxyl since her symptoms were primarily in the realm of metabolic rate, energy, and temperature production. (She had minimal gastrointestinal or skin symptoms that would have warranted T3.) At her follow-up visit six months later, Audrey's dose was 75 mcg of Levoxyl twice a day, and she felt like she was on the right dose! Her blood pressure was 116/70, and her pulse was 81 and regular. Her energy was good, and her weight had dropped 15 pounds. Audrey's periods were still heavy, however, and occurred only every 35 days. Her hands also remained cold. Her TSH was <0.004. I increased her dose slightly to 88 mcg twice daily and advised her to watch closely for any overdose symptoms. At that visit, she mentioned that she was planning a pregnancy soon and moving to Asheville, North Carolina.

Four months later, she called me from North Carolina to report that she was around six weeks pregnant and wanted to know what to do with her dose. I advised her to continue to take the dose that made her body work optimally and to consider seeking out a perinatologist to manage her thyroid dose during her pregnancy. A sonogram at 10 weeks showed a twin pregnancy displaying normal growth. Unfortunately, because of her low TSH, her obstetrician sent her to an endocrinologist, who convinced her to reduce her thyroid dose to achieve a "normal" TSH. Afraid to go against that recommendation, she did as was suggested, initially stopping her dose for a few days and then resuming 100 mcg once a day of levothyroxine. The result was that, at 15 weeks, Audrey was diagnosed as having twin fetal deaths in utero (FDIU). Her doctors identified no cause for the FDIU, but she and I both suspected that the sudden and significant drop in thyroid dose was the likely cause.

Three months later, Audrey came to northern Virginia from North Carolina to see me to get her thyroid rebalanced. This time, if she were to conceive again, she would not let anyone decrease her dose because of a low TSH value. She was back on 75 mcg of Levoxyl twice daily, and her hands were chilly. She was tired and constipated. As Audrey was clearly underdosed, I gave her a new dose titration schedule at that visit. She must have conceived about that time because 10 weeks later, she called to report that she was 10 weeks pregnant! About five weeks later, Audrey came to see me again on the dose of 100 mcg twice a day of levothyroxine because her hands remained chilly. She remained exhausted and cold, and we gave her another dose titration schedule to slowly increase her dose gradually by 25 mcg every two weeks to a maximum of 150 mcg of T4 twice daily. She also found a new and more open-minded obstetrician who would not insist that she had to have a normal TSH.

The following April, Audrey called to report that she had an uncomplicated full-term delivery of a healthy baby boy. We were both ecstatic! She had continued on a 125-mcg dose of levothyroxine in the morning, plus 100 mcg at noon throughout this pregnancy. She came to see me four months later, still on that dose, and she was now having symptoms of low thyroid. (Remember, pregnancy often reduces thyroid function in the mom.) Her symptoms were achy joints and puffy hands. Her pulse was 67, and her weight was 184 pounds. This time we decided to increase her T4 dose and perhaps add a little T3. Three months later – on 125 mcg of T4 twice a day plus 10 mcg of Cytomel in the morning plus 5 mcg in the afternoon – Audrey was once again feeling better with the resolution of the puffiness and achiness, good sleep, and no symptoms of overdose.

About 10 months later, she returned, now living in Pennsylvania, Audrey had stopped her Cytomel because it was making her jittery, and she was frequently missing her afternoon dose of T4. Consequently, she was tired and somewhat depressed. Audrey had read about Armour Thyroid and wanted to try it, so we gave her a titration schedule using Armour. Three months later, she returned for a follow-up visit, this time with her 20-month-old son! She was about 80% well, taking Armour Thyroid 90 mg in the morning, plus 60 mg at noon. Her TSH was .012, so I increased Audrey's dose a bit more, hoping to improve her persistent constipation and lack of energy. Both goals were achieved by increasing her dose to Armour Thyroid 120 mg twice daily.

What was most interesting during that visit was her remarkable baby boy. At age 20 months, after walking into my office from the reception area, where there were Lego blocks to play with, he confidently came over to the side of my desk. He carefully placed a small yellow Lego propeller on the corner of my desk. Then, he looked at me and clearly pronounced the word "fly"! I figured he was very intelligent for such a young age, and I quietly suspected that the thyroid stimulation that his mom had experienced during his gestation may have done good things for his brain development. What a fabulous outcome!!

"LYNNE"

Lynne, a part-time clerical worker, first came to see me at age 53, requesting hormone replacement. She had been referred to me by another long-term patient on HRT. Lynne was absolutely miserable with fatigue, low mood, hot flashes, foggy brain, dry vagina, dry skin, constipation, constant sweating, no libido, and disrupted sleep. She had been diagnosed and treated for breast cancer five years earlier and became menopausal at that time. Not only was she menopausal, but her oncologist had prescribed Femara, an aromatase inhibitor (an estrogen blocker) that made her estrogen deficiency symptoms even more severe.

Because of the diagnosis of breast cancer and the decades-long, nearly universal advice from the "experts" to avoid giving estrogen to breast cancer survivors, no prior doctor had been brave enough to give Lynne the hormones that would relieve her severe symptoms. In addition to her primary problem with menopause, she also had diagnoses of diabetes, high cholesterol, hypertension, and hypothyroidism treated by her internist with the standard dose of 100 mcg of Synthroid daily for the past 15 years. On exam, her blood pressure was 129/91, her pulse was 66, and her hands and feet were always cold. Lynne's TSH was normal, and her hemoglobin A1C was 6.8 on Glucophage (metformin). Her cholesterol on a statin drug was 165. Bone density evaluations showed a steady decrease in bone density during the years she was estrogen deficient.

I assessed that Lynne needed estrogen replacement – no progesterone was necessary since her uterus and ovaries were previously removed – and she also needed her thyroid dose adjusted. (Estrogen deficient women almost *never* have cold hands and feet unless they are also hypothyroid. The high cholesterol and diabetes both strongly suggested that she had a problem with her metabolic rate.

Since the idea of prescribing HRT to breast cancer patients was, to put it mildly, controversial, Lynne and I had an extensive discussion of the pros and cons and risks and benefits of that approach in her particular case. I gave her articles to read, including a 2002 article by Meurer and Lena[162] showing that postmenopausal patients who take HRT after being treated for breast cancer have significantly reduced mortality compared to those breast cancer patients who complied with the current dogma and avoided HRT. I encouraged Lynne to do as much research as she liked and to think about this before proceeding. In addition, I gave her a schedule to titrate her thyroid dose upward and switched her to Armour Thyroid from her current Synthroid, as she had dry skin and constipation, symptoms that suggested a T3 deficiency.

We had several phone calls to adjust her doses based on her symptoms, and I didn't see Lynne again until four years later. When she came to see me, she was back on Synthroid at 100 mcg daily. She said she had indigestion with the Armour Thyroid and discontinued it. She had also stopped her estrogen because her 88-year-old aunt had been diagnosed with ovarian cancer. (Interestingly, the data do not show a consistent correlation between estrogen replacement and ovarian cancer. Nevertheless, fear remains a strong motivator.)

Lynne's vital signs included a blood pressure of 124/84, a pulse of 64, and a weight of 190 pounds at a height of 5' 4 3/4 ". She had returned because she wanted to regain the benefits that she had experienced previously. Her TSH was still normal at 2.29, and her hemoglobin A1C was 7.5.

We again discussed the pros and cons of HRT and resumed estrogen. This time, we also increased her dose of Synthroid since she was clearly underdosed and Armour had given her heartburn. We fine-tuned her doses of estrogen and thyroid over the next several years, and at the three-year mark, Lynne was feeling very well with good energy and sleep, taking 150 mcg of Synthroid in the morning, plus 125 mcg at noon, with.45 mg of Premarin daily. Her weight was down to 185, her pulse was 61, and her blood pressure was 115/68. Her TSH was, as expected, down to <0.005. In addition, the bone loss she had been experiencing on Femara had stabilized.

Since then, Lynne continued to feel very well on these doses with occasional minor adjustments. Her last visit with me occurred about two weeks before I retired. At that time, she was still feeling very well, her weight was down to 155 pounds, and she no longer needed most of her diabetes meds! She definitely falls into the "better living with hormones" category and demonstrates that properly treating underlying hypothyroidism can benefit other conditions such as diabetes! That's a win-win in my book…and in hers as well!

"TRUDY"

Trudy was a 45-year-old consultant with a history of depression and stomach problems. She was referred to me by her friend, a patient of mine. Four years earlier, she suddenly became tired, achy, anxious and depressed, foggy-brained, and had difficulty finding words or remembering things. She also had developed very dry, brittle nails and dry, cracking feet. Trudy had been hospitalized at NIH for seven months as they tried to diagnose the cause of her illness. They had given her 12 treatments of ECT (electroconvulsive therapy) for treatment-resistant depression and three sleep studies to evaluate her disrupted sleep patterns. She had also tried acupuncture and physical therapy.

Trudy reported that she frequently napped and was usually so cold that she often wore a coat at home. Her hair was falling out in clumps, and she had gained 60 pounds in the past five years. She was previously a world traveler and was now on disability due to her illness. She also took daily Topamax, Prozac, Ambien, Prevacid and ½ of a Tylenol PM tablet. In addition, Trudy had a hormonal IUD called Mirena inserted to control her heavy periods. (In general, progesterone IUDs are a terrible idea in someone who is very hypothyroid since they can make the patient suicidal.) Her vital signs included a blood pressure of 125/88 and a pulse of 75. At 5' 7", she weighed 245 pounds. Her TSH was, of course, "normal" at 2.184, which made it impossible for all the medical experts at NIH to see the classic and severe symptoms of hypothyroidism that were clearly visible in front of their expert – albeit blindfolded – eyes.

With all these apparent signs of severe thyroid deficiency, I recommended that Trudy start treatment. After discussing the pros/cons and what to expect, she began a titration schedule using Armour Thyroid. Four months later, at her first follow-up visit, taking 90 mg of Armour Thyroid twice a day, Trudy reported that she was feeling slightly better; her energy had improved, and her feet were warmer. She was no longer on psychiatric medications and was doing well without them! Trudy was pleased that her periods had disappeared on the Mirena IUD, the normal response to the progesterone in that product. Her weight and vital signs were unchanged, but she was no longer gaining weight. Because she was not yet "well," we gave her a new titration dose, increasing the dose a bit more.

Her next visit occurred four months later, and her weight was down to 214 pounds! Her pulse was 85 and regular, and her blood pressure was 126/88. Unfortunately, Trudy had increased her dose more than she was advised and was now taking 240 mg of Armour Thyroid twice daily (4 grains twice a day). On this dose, her hair loss had finally stopped, her skin was no longer dry, and she was no longer achy. Happily, Trudy was not feeling or showing any signs of overdose symptoms despite not following directions and increasing her dose higher than we had planned. Because she appeared well and had no evidence that the dose was excessive, I allowed Trudy to continue that dose for a few more months and decided to reassess her status later. We again discussed the risks of overdose and the need to monitor her pulse daily.

About a month later, Trudy called, stating that her pulse was up to 104, and she wanted to know what to do. She was advised to stop her dose until her pulse normalized, which it did with no adverse effect. When the symptoms of low thyroid began to return, and she started feeling drowsy, we resumed a smaller dose of Armour Thyroid. She ended up on 120 mg of Armour Thyroid twice a day (2 grains, twice a day), which was half of her last dose, and she remained on that dose for the next several years with good resolution of almost all of her initial symptoms.

About a year later, Trudy had a fall and sustained a concussion. She had some neurologic deficits from that fall, and a neurologist managed those. Though she was still on the same dose of Armour Thyroid 120 mg twice a day, she started to have a recurrence of some of her symptoms, including weight gain back up to 262 pounds, dry skin, hair loss, fatigue, and fogginess. Her pulse was 71, and her blood pressure was 122/87. Due to the return of those symptoms, I again advised her to increase the dose a little bit more with a new titration schedule and advised her to continue to watch closely for any signs of excess thyroid. But because Trudy then had a "physical" with another doctor who did a TSH test that came back low, she decided to stay on her current dose of Armour Thyroid 120 mg twice daily. She did increase her dose again the following year up to Armour Thyroid 180 mg twice a day (3 grains twice a day) due to the persistence of her fatigue, weight gain, poor sleep, hair loss, and cold feet, which once again helped relieve her symptoms. On that dose Trudy was once again well.

This case illustrates two things exceptionally well. First, it shows how blinded even the best and brightest physicians have become by their irrational belief that blood tests are somehow more valid than what is actually going on clinically with the patient. Again, in the words of Osler and Woodward after him: *"If you just ask the patient, they will usually tell you what is wrong!"* Trudy was perfectly capable of reporting her symptoms, which would lead any first-year medical student to the correct diagnosis. Still, all the "experts" at the National Institutes of Health couldn't help her because they trusted their TSH blood test over what their eyes could see, and their ears could hear. A massive amount of money was spent by these "experts" going around in diagnostic circles in a fancy hospital setting only to fail to arrive at the correct diagnosis.

The other lesson illustrated here is that patients sometimes don't follow directions perfectly. Fortunately, thyroid hormone, unlike, for example, insulin, is a very forgiving hormone. You need to take too much for a long time to get into serious trouble. Consequently, in this and the large majority of such cases, no serious adverse event occurred, and Trudy's elevated pulse returned to normal relatively quickly after stopping her dose. But that may not always be the case.

I encourage patients to follow directions and communicate with your physicians. And if your physician doesn't listen and isn't helping you get well, it's time to find one who will!

As for my fellow doctors, make sure you educate your patients and explain the possible consequences of taking too much thyroid. Limiting the number of refills you give the patient is one option, so they will quickly run out of medication if they take more than what is prescribed. You might also consider having the patient sign a contract for care at the first visit, explaining that their care will be terminated if they fail to follow your directions. Again, this may seem harsh, but patients sometimes need that extra layer of motivation so that they proceed safely with their thyroid dose titration and don't decide to go rogue and get themselves into trouble.

"ELIZABETH"

Being a world-class opera singer, Elizabeth was probably my most famous patient. She was referred to me by her sister, a voice instructor, who was also my patient. Elizabeth first came to my office at age 56 and had already started on estrogen replacement 18 months earlier. She was generally quite healthy, though she had many classic symptoms of low thyroid function. Her medicines included Cymbalta, Arthrotec, metformin, and .05 mg Vivelle Dot estrogen patches. Her symptoms of low thyroid included hair thinning, low energy, weight gain, low mood, foggy brain, dry skin, food cravings, constipation, cold intolerance, poor sleep, and occasional hot flashes. Her pulse was 68, her blood pressure was 102/65, and at 5'6", she weighed 169 pounds. Her TSH was 1.172, perfectly normal.

Elizabeth continued her HRT, and since she had symptoms suggesting a deficiency of both T4 and T3, she started on a titration schedule of Armour Thyroid. Even on Armour Thyroid 30 mg twice daily, she was feeling better energy and mood, and her thinking was sharper! Elizabeth felt so good that she was able to get off the Cymbalta! However, she did indicate that her appetite was noticeably increased, so we discussed possibly replacing some of the Armour with some T4 to decrease the appetite stimulation. Elizabeth opted to stay with Armour, and at her 4-month follow-up visit, she was taking Armour Thyroid 90 mg twice a day and was continuing to improve but was still having some hair and constipation issues, and her weight was up 10 pounds! She had also developed more hot flashes that I suspected were due to increased clearance of her Vivelle Dot .05 mg patches, a small dose for an active young woman. Her pulse remained normal at 65. Her TSH was now .008.

We increased Elizabeth's estrogen dose to .1 mg of Vivelle Dot patch and replaced some of her Armour with levothyroxine because she felt a little jittery after her morning coffee. Later, we also increased her thyroid dose by 30 mg (½ grain). She was on 60 mg (1 grain) of Armour in the morning and 200 mcg (2 grains) of levothyroxine at noon. Interestingly, after two years of this management, Elizabeth mentioned that her voice had improved! She also started losing a bit of weight, and her energy was excellent! Sadly, about two years later, some of her symptoms began to return, including afternoon fatigue, skin dryness, and cold intolerance, and she had gained 7 pounds. Therefore, I slowly increased her Armour and T4 to a total dose of 60 mg (1 grain) of Armour Thyroid twice a day plus 50 mcg of T4 in the morning plus 200 mcg in the afternoon. Happily, on this dose, Elizabeth regained her previous level of wellness.

I found it interesting that several other of my professional singer patients mentioned that thyroid replacement improved their singing voices. Perhaps the International Union of Voice Coaches should be made aware of this effect!

"EMILY"

Emily was a very intelligent self-employed programmer with a very complicated thyroid history. She first came to see me in 2016 at the age of 51. She lived several hours away from my office. At her initial visit, she brought a 16-page document that outlined her complex and very distressing history of thyroid "management." She was currently on thyroid medication but knew her current dose was inadequate. Her goal was to hopefully have me increase her current thyroid replacement dose to achieve the wellness level she previously enjoyed when taking 100 mcg of Cytomel three times per day (12 grains)! Emily's current dose was 175 mcg of levothyroxine plus 25 mcg of generic T3 (2 3/4 grains).

To make a very long history short, Emily's hypothyroidism symptoms first appeared after the birth of her second child in 1987. But because her labs were normal, no thyroid hormone was prescribed. Then in 1994, Emily developed a strep abscess in her neck associated with a temperature of 105.9. A CT scan at that time showed a multinodular goiter. She was hospitalized for 24 days, spending the first 10 days in the ICU. She was not expected to survive that ordeal. At that time, her thyroid tests were normal, so thyroid was still not prescribed.

The following year, Emily saw a dermatologist to evaluate her hair loss. He suspected hypothyroidism and therefore wisely referred her to an endocrinologist, but again, her labs were "normal," so she was not offered treatment. Shortly after that, a urologist referred her to endocrinology with the same presumed diagnosis, and sadly the patient got the same response. Then, in 1998, her ENT also referred her to an endocrinologist for thyroid management, and according to the patient's notes, "He walked me over to the clinic and made sure that they gave me an appointment."

At that time, Emily was finally given a small amount of Synthroid to "shrink her goiter" and was later switched to 100 mcg of Cytomel three times a day – a very high dose! Most of her symptoms resolved. She then developed some problems swallowing, so she had a total thyroidectomy in 2001 to treat her enlarged thyroid. Her dose was later reduced to 300 mg (5 grains) of Armour daily by a UVA endocrinologist because she considered the Cytomel dose, which was working well for her, to be "toxic."

It's interesting that Emily also had a very strong history of hypothyroidism in many family members, including her father, who "was in a coma and later died due to complications of hypothyroidism." (The medical term for a coma due to severe hypothyroidism is myxedema coma.) Most had a delayed diagnosis of their thyroid problems due to their normal thyroid tests.

Despite being on some thyroid replacement after her thyroidectomy, in 2014, Emily was admitted to the hospital with severe heart failure due to myxedema. Her ejection fraction at the time of that admission was 7%. (Normal is 50% to 75%.) During that time, she had also experienced massive dysfunctional uterine bleeding that required multiple blood transfusions. A D&C was performed and revealed no cancer at that time. She was on 10 mg of Provera twice a day to prevent the recurrence of bleeding. Her ejection fraction at her first visit was still sub-optimal at 33%.

Other than persistent moderate cardiac failure due to suboptimal thyroid dosing, Emily's other symptoms included fatigue, significant swelling and edema, respiratory congestion, increased weight, dry skin patches, cold intolerance, hair loss, achiness, fragile nails, foggy brain, hypertension, and constipation. In addition, her tendency to have very heavy periods was controlled with a large daily dose of progesterone. Her current medications were Lisinopril, Carvedilol, generic Provera, Bumex (a diuretic), Loratadine, a Proair inhaler, a daily low-dose aspirin, and thyroid medication. She also had multiple drug allergies and took multiple vitamin and mineral supplements. Emily listed two GP's, three cardiologists, one endocrinologist, two Ob-Gyn's, one urologist, and one chiropractor on her medical history sheet. Her vital signs at her first visit were a blood pressure of 116/84, a pulse of 103 (after a drive of several hours), and she was 5'6" and weighed 324 pounds.

Emily's dose of 175 mcg of T4 plus 25 mcg of Cytomel once a day (2.75 grains total) was clearly inadequate, and it was clear from her detailed history and presentation that 1) she needed more thyroid, and 2) she did well with T3. But I was reluctant to go up too rapidly with her dose. Therefore, we first tried increasing her dose up to

120 mg (2 grains) of natural desiccated thyroid twice a day, and I asked her to call me in three to four weeks with a status report. We chose to use WP Thyroid at that time instead of Armour. Emily felt more energetic in the afternoons since the new dose was evenly split between morning and noon dosing. However, she had more hair loss, worsening skin, and a poor appetite, all signs that she needed an increase in her dose, especially more T3. Her basal temperature remained from 95.5 to 96.3. Of course, she had no symptoms of overdose. We then increased her dose to 150 mg (2 ½ grains) of WP Thyroid twice a day. This improved her hair and bowel function, but she still felt tired and cold, classic symptoms of low T4. So, we increased her morning and noon doses by 30 mg (½ grain) every three weeks.

On 180 mg (3 grains) of WP Thyroid in the morning plus 120 mg (2 grains) at noon and 250 mcg of T4 twice a day, Emily was starting to feel better, and her cardiac ejection fraction was now up to 42%. She was able to discontinue her Bumex diuretic since her heart function was improving, and she could decrease her progesterone dose by half. Emily still had some symptoms – including hair loss, dry skin, and poor appetite – so we added more WP Thyroid. She improved somewhat but still didn't feel entirely well. Since she showed no signs of overdose, we continued to increase her dose slowly and cautiously, adding more WP Thyroid.

In November 2017, Emily developed atrial fibrillation and was admitted to a local hospital. I advised her to stop her entire dose, to allow the dose to flush out of her system. The rhythm quickly normalized, and she was discharged in two days. Her husband mentioned that he suspected she had accidentally taken a double dose of her WP Thyroid by mistake before that episode occurred. She reported that her pulse had been normal before this episode. After discussing with Emily what dose she had been taking when this happened, it became evident that she had been adjusting her dose from time to time on her own and had not consistently communicated with me about those changes. I asked Emily to make no further changes on her own and to remain on 210 mg (3½ grains) of WP Thyroid twice daily, with only 150 mcg of T4 twice a day. This was still a very large dose, but less than she had been taking recently. She remained stable and well on that dose for the next couple of years. (Interestingly, this dose was almost equivalent to the dose of Cytomel that had made her well at the onset of her saga.)

Unfortunately, two years later, Emily had another health crisis requiring hospitalization, which her discharging physician described as due to *"septic shock and heart failure exacerbation."* She was treated with antibiotics, diuretics, and IV levothyroxine and somehow miraculously recovered. At this point, I realized that it would be in Emily's best interest – and probably mine as well – to have her thyroid needs managed by someone who was closer geographically to her and better able to monitor her progress closely. I've found that doing long-distance thyroid management is never ideal and is not something that I generally recommend to patients with hypothyroidism. Emily understood that and transferred her care to her local endocrinologist. I hope that she is doing well under his care.

"ROBERTA"

Roberta was the owner of a local family martial arts facility and a daycare center. At age 37, she sought, as she said, "an open-minded physician to better assess possible thyroid/hormonal issues. I've always had low thyroid symptoms, but never low enough to be diagnosed." She had been referred to me by a local chiropractor. Her history included three live births and four miscarriages, symptoms suggesting PCOS, elevated cholesterol, and a need to take extreme measures to lose weight. All of Roberta's pregnancies were complicated by hypertension, and she wanted to be in optimal health before attempting another pregnancy. She was taking no medication but was on many vitamin and herbal supplements and trying to follow a ketogenic diet.

Roberta's symptoms of low thyroid included weight issues, hair loss, anxiety, foggy brain, low energy, cravings, tendency to have increased blood pressure and high cholesterol, puffiness, a scalloped tongue, dry skin, and constipation. Her labs values included a TSH of 1.09 and cholesterol of 221. At this first visit, at a height of 5'8", she weighed 244 pounds, her pulse was 91, and her blood pressure was 139/102. Her normal blood pressure was around 130/85.

Since she had symptoms of both low T3 and low T4, Roberta started on a titration schedule using NP Thyroid in the mornings and T4 for her noon dose. She was taking 90 mg (1½ grains) of NP Thyroid in the morning and 150 mcg of T4 at noon at the time of her follow-up visit five months later. Roberta had been on that dose for about three months and reported that her energy had improved by about a third. Unfortunately, she forgot to take some doses over the holidays, gained about 10 pounds, and had persistent hair loss. But all the other news was positive. Roberta's scalloped tongue had normalized shortly after starting thyroid replacement. She no longer needed 10 to 12 hours of sleep each night, and her anxiety was somewhat reduced. Her pulse was 80, and she had no signs or symptoms of overdose.

Since some of her symptoms remained, I gave Roberta a new titration schedule with further increases in both the NP and T4 doses, increasing by 30 mg (½ grain) every three weeks with repeated instructions to watch carefully for any signs of overdose. At her next visit six months later, she was on 120 mg of NP Thyroid in the morning and 300 mcg of T4 at noon. Now, her hair was growing back, and her focus was much improved. Her anxiety had disappeared, and she felt energetic after eight hours of sleep. Her bowel movements were normal, her weight was now down to 212 pounds, and her cholesterol had dropped to 206. Roberta was very happy with this dose and continued to have no signs or symptoms of overdose, so we stayed on this dose, despite her predictably low TSH of <0.005.

However, she returned six months later with increased fatigue, a slight tremor, an increased appetite, weight gain back up to 245, and a pulse of 109. Her average resting pulse at home was 84. Roberta was not in acute distress by any stretch of the imagination. Still, I suspected that her tremor, increased appetite, and weight gain were the effects of slightly too much T3, and the increased pulse was evidence of too much T4. We reduced her dose by a third, to NP Thyroid 60 mg twice daily plus T4 100 mcg twice a day. That change was perfect. Roberta felt well; the symptoms of excess thyroid resolved promptly, and her pulse now averaged 76. In addition, one month later, she reported having a positive pregnancy test! I referred her to an open-minded obstetrician and encouraged her to continue this dose as long as it kept her body working well!

"KELLY"

Kelly, a homemaker who previously worked as a health promotions coordinator at a local women's college, first came to me at age 56 for hormonal management. She was diagnosed with hypothyroidism due to Hashimoto's thyroiditis. She had been prescribed 30 mg (½ grain) of Armour Thyroid three times a day (a total of 90 mg or 1.5 grains) by a local, relatively open-minded endocrinologist. She also used vaginal estrogen to control severe vaginal dryness, but with minimal success. Her last period was two years earlier. Kelly's most significant issues were hair loss, persistent vaginal dryness, frequent urinary tract infections since the onset of menopause, and low libido.

Upon examination, I noted that Kelly was a thin woman with temporal balding and cool hands, and at 5' 5", she weighed 110 pounds. Her pulse was 75, and her blood pressure was 126/80. Her most recent TSH was normal at 0.49. My initial thoughts were 1) that she needed a much more aggressive approach to treating her estrogen deficiency and 2) that the high T3/T4 ratio in the Armour Thyroid was likely making her hair loss worse.

Here are some tips about estrogen replacement. Menopause hits thin women much harder than heavier women since thin women have no fat storage of estrogen. As a result, thin women usually need higher doses of estrogen to resolve menopausal symptoms. Also, thin women tend to have much more bone loss than their heavier counterparts, which needs to be addressed. Treating only her vaginal dryness and allowing her to have unchecked bone loss was clearly not the best or most responsible approach to treating Kelly's estrogen deficiency.

We continued the estrogen vaginal cream and added full systemic estrogen and progesterone replacement. Hoping to fix Kelly's hair loss, we switched her to just levothyroxine, starting at 100 mcg twice a day and slowly titrating the dose upward. The goals of the therapy were to stop her hair loss, help her achieve softer skin, cure her blepharitis (inflamed/infected eyelashes and lids), reduce her gastric reflux, entirely fix the vaginal and urinary tract issues, warm up her feet, and give her good energy.

Three months later, Kelly was taking 150 mcg of Levoxyl in the morning, plus 100 mcg at noon – along with her 0.1 mg estradiol patch and 100 mg of progesterone by mouth at bedtime – she had partial improvement. Her vaginal issues and libido were significantly better. She had some improvement in her hair and skin symptoms, as well as her blepharitis. Her pulse was 68, and she had no symptoms of thyroid overdose. She struggled with cold feet and hands and used a hot water bottle to warm her feet every night.

Consequently, we increased her dose slowly and added a little Armour Thyroid back into her treatment because her eyes remained dry. Approximately six months after her first visit, she had gotten up to 150 mcg of Levoxyl twice a day, plus 30 mg of NP Thyroid twice daily, along with her full dose of HRT. She was essentially cured, with a good resolution of all of her symptoms. And, no surprise, her final TSH claimed otherwise!

APPENDIX C: RESOURCES

Links to resources are also available online at the book's website, https://www.doctorhurlock.com.

RECOMMENDED BOOKS

Barnes BO, Galton L. *Hypothyroidism: The Unsuspected Illness.* New York: Harper & Row; 1976. 286 p.

Barnes BO, Barnes CW. *Solved: The Riddle of Heart Attacks.* 6th edition. Fort Collins, CO: Robinson Press, Inc.; 1984. 74 p. Available from The Broda Barnes Foundation; Trumbull, CT; at https://brodabarnes.org/bookstore.htm.

Starr M. *Hypothyroidism Type 2.* Columbia, MO: Mark Starr Trust; 2005. 242 p.

Skinner GRB. *Diagnosis and Management of Hypothyroidism.* Biggleswade, UK: Watkiss Studios, Ltd.; 2003. 199 p.

Bluming A, Tavris C. *Estrogen Matters.* New York; Little, Brown Spark; 2018. 245 p.

Gaby, Alan MD. *Preventing and Reversing Osteoporosis.* Prima Publishing, 1994. 290 p.

Holick MA. *The Vitamin D Solution: A 3-step Strategy to Cure Our Most Common Health Problems.* Paperback, illustrated edition. NYC: Plume, Penguin Books, Inc; 2011. 336 p.

NATURAL DESICCATED THYROID (NDT) DRUGS

Armour Thyroid - www.armourthyroid.com

NP Thyroid - www.npthyroid.com

Nature-Throid - www.naturethroid.com

WP Thyroid - www.wpthyroid.com

LEVOTHYROXINE (T4) DRUGS

Euthyrox Levothyroxine Tablets - www.provellpharma.com/euthyrox-us

Levoxyl Levothyroxine Tablets - www.pfizer.com/products/product-detail/Levoxyl

Synthroid Levothyroxine Tablets - www.synthroid.com

Tirosint Levothyroxine Capsules - tirosint.com

Tirosint-SOL Levothyroxine Oral Solution - tirosintsol.com

Unithroid Levothyroxine Tablets - www.unithroid.com

LIOTHYRONINE (T3) DRUG

Cytomel - www.pfizermedicalinformation.com/en-us/patient/cytomel

LOW-COST ONLINE PHARMACIES

Honeybee Health – honeybeehealth.com

Cost Plus Drug Company - costplusdrugs.com

DISCOUNT PRICES AND COUPONS FOR DRUGS

(Often cheaper than insurance copays)

GoodRx.com – www.goodrx.com

SingleCare – www.singlecare.com

FIND DOCTORS

ThyroidChange Recommended Doctor List - www.thyroidchange.org/patient-recommended-doctor-list-us.html

PalomaHealth – www.palomahealth.com

Get Real Thyroid - getrealthyroid.com/find-a-thyroid-doctor.html

American College for Advancement in Medicine — Integrative Physician Finder - acam.site-ym.com/search/custom.asp?id=1758v

Lifescript's Doctors Who Treat or Diagnose Hormonal Imbalance - www.lifescript.com/doctor-directory/condition/h-hormonal-imbalance.aspx

The American College for Advancement in Medicine's Physician+Link - Integrative Doctor Database - acam.site-ym.com/search/custom.asp?id=1758

The International College of Integrative Medicine's ICIM Member Search - www.icimed.com/member_search.php

American Board of Integrative Holistic Medicine Database - www.aihm.org/search/custom.asp?id=4620

American Association of Naturopathic Physicians - Find a Naturopathic Doctor Database - naturopathic.org/search/custom.asp?id=5613

OTHER RESOURCES

The Optimal Treatment for Hypothyroidism – by the late Dr. John Lowe DC – www.tpauk.com/main/article/the-optimal-treatment-for-hypothyroidism-by-the-late-dr-john-lowe-dc/

Dr. John Lowe's Thyroid Science - drlowe.com/thyroidscience

National Academy of Hypothyroidism – www.NAhypothyroidism.org

Gold Care – www.goldcare.com

Association of American Physicians and Surgeons – www.AAPSonline.org

International Association for Premenstrual Disorders – www.IAPMD.org

PubMed – www.Pubmed.gov

Science Direct – www.ScienceDirect.com

Theravive – www.theravive.com

Thyroid Advisor – www.thyroidadvisor.com

Thyroid Change – www.thyroidchange.org

The Wedge – www.jointhewedge.com

Natural Thyroid Guide – www.naturalthyroidguide.com

Mary Shomon / Thyroid Patient Advocate – www.mary-shomon.com

ABOUT THE AUTHOR

After graduating Magna cum Laude and Phi Beta Kappa from Duke University, Donna Hurlock earned her medical degree from the University of Maryland, Baltimore, and did her internship and residency at the Washington Hospital Center. She was board-certified as an obstetrician/gynecologist in 1985 and practiced obstetrics/gynecology in a group practice until 1988 when she opened her practice, "Donna G Hurlock, MD, PC," later renamed the Women's Hormone Center of Northern Virginia, PC. In her solo private practice, Dr. Hurlock focused on gynecology and hormonal health, including managing thyroid hormone replacement for thousands of women.

Dr. Hurlock has been a NAMS (North American Menopause Society) Certified Menopause Practitioner since 2000. She is a member of the American Association of Physicians and Surgeons and the Florida Medical Association, and a past member of the Board of Advisors for the Physicians Committee for Responsible Medicine in Washington, DC.

Dr. Hurlock's peer-reviewed journal publications include:

Barnard ND, Scialli AR, Bertron P, Hurlock D, Edmonds B. "Acceptability of a Therapeutic Low-Fat, Vegan Diet in Premenopausal Women," *J of Nutrition Ed*, vol 32, #6, Nov/Dec 2000.

Barnard ND, Scialli AR, Bertron P, Hurlock D. "Effectiveness of a low-fat vegetarian diet in altering serum lipids in healthy premenopausal women," *Amer J of Cardiol*, vol 85, Apr 2000

Barnard ND, Scialli AR, Hurlock D, Bertron P. "Diet and sex-hormone binding globulin, dysmenorrhea, and premenstrual symptoms," *Obstet Gynecol*, 95(2): 245-50, Feb 2000.

Dr. Hurlock has authored various guides and publications including *The Truth about Estrogen*, and articles in many newspapers, journals, websites, and media outlets, including *OB-GYN News* and *PCRM Update* among others.

Dr. Hurlock has made a number of television and radio news and interview appearances discussing hormonal and reproductive health for location and national outlets, including National Public Radio. She's also been interviewed/quoted for articles in *Cosmopolitan Magazine, Discover Magazine, Better Nutrition Magazine, WebMD*, and many newspapers and magazines.

Dr. Hurlock has been a featured expert in numerous books, including *The Menopause Thyroid Solution*, and *Guidelines from Experts in Thyroid Disease Diagnosis and Management of Hypothyroidism in Women.*

Dr. Hurlock has lectured on hormonal and reproductive health issues to numerous groups, including the American Association of University Women and the Physicians Committee for Responsible Medicine.

Dr. Hurlock retired from private medical practice in 2021, and now lives in Florida, where she pursues her passions for patient advocacy, boating, civic volunteering, and living the Florida lifestyle.

CITATIONS

Clickable links to the book's citations are available online at the book's website, https://www.doctorhurlock.com.

[1] Hart FD, MacLagan NF. Oral thyroxine in treatment of myxoedema. *British Medical Journal.* 1950 Mar 4; 1(4652): 512-518. Available from: https://www.bmj.com/content/1/4652/512

[2] Thyroidadvisor.com [Internet]. Armour thyroid and Synthroid complete overview. 2016 Jul 29 [Cited 2021 Feb 22]. Available from: https://thyroidadvisor.com/armour-thyroid-synthroid-complete-overview/.

[3] Hennessey J (Division of Endocrinology, Department of Medicine, Beth Israel Deaconess Medical Center, Boston, MA, USA), Espaillat R (Abbvie Inc., North Chicago, IL, USA). Current evidence for the treatment of hypothyroidism with levothyroxine/levotriiodothyronine combination therapy versus levothyroxine monotherapy. *International Journal of Clinical Practice* (John Wiley & Sons Ltd.) [Internet]. 2018 Feb; 72(2): e13062. Available from: https://onlinelibrary.wiley.com/doi/10.1111/ijcp.13062/.

[4] American Medical Association, Council on Pharmacy and Chemistry. *Useful Drugs.* 6th edition. Chicago, IL: American Medical Association; 1923. 171 p.

[5] Duman D (Dept of Cardiology, Haydarpasa Numune Training and Research Hospital, Istanbul, Turkey), Sahin S, Esertas K, Demirtunc R. Simvastatin improves endothelial function in patents with subclinical hypothyroidism. *Heart Vessels* [Internet]. 2007 Mar; 22(2): 88-93. Available from: https://pubmed.ncbi.nlm.nih.gov/17390202/.

[6] Barnes BO, Galton L. *Hypothyroidism: the Unsuspected Illness.* New York: Harper & Row; 1976. 286 p.

[7] Cooper D (Chair, Endocrinology and Metabolism, Johns Hopkins University, Baltimore, MD, USA). Written personal communication. 2012 Sep 6.

[8] Starr M. *Hypothyroidism Type 2.* Columbia, MO: Mark Starr Trust; 2005. 242 p.

[9] Blum A, Behl M, Birnbaum L, Diamond M, Phillips A, Singla V, Sipes N, Stapleton H, Venier M. Organophosphate ester flame retardants: Are they a regrettable substitution for polybrominated diphenyl ethers? *Environmental Science & Technology Letters* (American Chemical Society Publications) [Internet]. 2019 Oct 21; 6(11): 638-649. Available from: https://pubs.acs.org/doi/10.1021/acs.estlett.9b00582.

[10] Moccia RD, Leatherland JF, Sonstegard RA. Quantitative interlake comparison of thyroid pathology in Great Lakes coho (Oncorhynchus kisutch) and chinook (Oncorhynchus tschawaytscha) salmon [comparative study]. Cancer research [Internet]. 1981 Jun; 41(6): 2200-10. Available from: https://pubmed.ncbi.nlm.nih.gov/7237420/.

[11] BTF-thyroid.org [Internet]. Harrogate, UK: British Thyroid Foundation; 2022. Thyroid disease in dogs and cats [Cited 2022 July 30]. Available from: https://www.btf-thyroid.org/thyroid-disease-in-dogs-and-cats.

[12] Hodis HN (Atherosclerosis Research Unit, University of Southern California, Los Angeles, CA), Mack WJ, Henderson

VW, Shoupe D, Budoff MJ, Hwang-Levine J, Li Y, Feng M, Dustin L, Kono N, Stanczyk FZ, Selzer RH, Azen SP, et al., for the ELITE Research Group. Vascular effect of early versus late postmenopausal treatment with estradiol. *New England Journal of Medicine* [Internet]. 2016 Mar 31; 374: 1221-31. Available from: https://www.nejm.org/doi/full/10.1056/nejmoa1505241/.

[13] Hodis HN, Mack WJ, Lobo RA, Shoupe D, Sevanian A, Mahrer PR, Selzer RH, Liu CR, Liu CH, Azen SP, Estrogen in the Prevention of Atherosclerosis Trial Research Group. Estrogen in the prevention of atherosclerosis. A randomized, double-blind, placebo-controlled trial [clinical trial]. *Annals of Internal Medicine* [Internet]. 2001 Dec 4; 135(11): 939-53. Available from: https://pubmed.ncbi.nlm.nih.gov/11730394/.

[14] Barnes BO, Barnes CW. *Solved: The Riddle of Heart Attacks.* 6th edition. Fort Collins, CO: Robinson Press, Inc.; 1984. 74 p. Available from: The Broda Barnes Foundation; Trumbull, CT; at https://brodabarnes.org/bookstore.htm.

[15] Writing Group for the Women's Health Initiative Investigators. Risks and Benefits of Estrogen Plus Progestin in Healthy Postmenopausal Women: Principal Results From the Women's Health Initiative Randomized Controlled Trial. *JAMA.* 2002;288(3):321–333. doi:10.1001/jama.288.3.321 https://jamanetwork.com/journals/jama/fullarticle/195120/.

[16] Bluming A, Tavris C. *Estrogen Matters.* New York; Little, Brown Spark; 2018. 245 p.

[17] Meurer LN, Lena S. Cancer recurrence and mortality in women using hormone replacement therapy: meta-analysis. *Journal of Family Practice* [Internet]. 2002 Dec; 51(12): 1056-62. Available from: https://pubmed.ncbi.nlm.nih.gov/12540332.

[18] Coelingh Bennink HJT, Verhoeven C, Dutman AE, Thijssen J (The Netherlands). The use of high-dose estrogens for the treatment of breast cancer [review]. *Maturitas* [Internet]. 2017; 95: 11-23. Available from:

https://sciencedirect.com/science/article/pii/SO378512216302833

[19] Bluming A, Tavris C. *Estrogen Matters.* New York; Little, Brown Spark; 2018. 245 p.

[20] NYU Long Island School of Medicine [Internet]. 2022: NYU Langone Health. MD Course Descriptions; [Cited 2019 Sep 25]. Available from: https://medli.nyu.edu/education/md-degree/md-curriculum/course-descriptions.

[21] SleepDr, The Sleep Blog [Internet]. Encino, CA: Advanced Sleep Medicine Services, Inc. 2020; 1994-2022. How much will a sleep study cost me? 2018 [Cited 2020 Nov 2]. Available from: https://www.sleepdr.com/the-sleep-blog/how-much-will-a-sleep-study-cost-me/.

[22] Millman RP, Bevilacqua J, Peterson DD, Pack AI. Central sleep apnea in hypothyroidism [case report]. *American Review of Respiratory Diseases* [Internet]. 1983 Apr; 127(4): 504-7. Available from: https://pubmed.ncbi.nlm.nih.gov/6838058/.

[23] Kittle WM, Chaudhary BA. Sleep apnea and hypothyroidism [review]. *Southern Medical Journal* [Internet]. 1988 Nov; 81(11): 1421-5. Available from: https://pubmed.ncbi.nlm.nih.gov/3055327/.

[24] Hira HS (Pulmonary Medicine & Sleep Centre, New Delhi, India), Sibal L. Sleep apnea syndrome among patients with hypothyroidism. *Journal of the Association of Physicians India* [Internet]. 1999 Jun; 47(6): 615-8. Available from: https://pubmed.ncbi.nlm.nih.gov/10999160/.

[25] Grunstein RR (Dept. of Thoracic Medicine, Royal Prince Alfred Hospital, Sydney, Australia), Sullivan CE (no affiliation listed). Sleep apnea and hypothyroidism: mechanisms and management [case report]. *American Journal of Medicine* [Internet]. 1988 Dec; 85(6): 775-9. Available from: https://pubmed.ncbi.nlm.nih.gov/3057899/.

[26] Gaby, Alan MD. Preventing and Reversing Osteoporosis. Prima Publishing, 1994 https://www.youtube.com/watch?v=x9Hz9pXb1TE.

[27] Tuchendler D, Bolanowski M. The influence of thyroid dysfunction on bone metabolism. *Thyroid Res.* [Internet] 2014 Dec 20;7(1):12. doi: 10.1186/s13044-014-0012-0. PMID: 25648501; PMCID: PMC4314789. Available from: https://www.ncbi.nlm.nih.gov/pmc/articles/PMC4314789/.

[28] Williams GR, Bassett JHD. Thyroid diseases and bone health [review]. *Journal of Endocrinology Investigations* [Internet]. 2018 Jan; 41(1): 99-109. Available from: https://pubmed.ncbi.nlm.nih.gov/28853052/.

[29] Gold HK, Spann JF, Braunwald E. Effect of alterations in the thyroid state on the intrinsic contractile properties of isolated rat skeletal muscle. *Journal of Clinical Investigations* [Internet]. 11970 Apr; 49(4): 849-54. Available from: https://pubmed.ncbi.nlm.nih.gov/5443184/.

[30] Flaim KE, Li JB, Jefferson LS. Effects of thyroxine on protein turnover in rat skeletal muscle. *American Journal of Physiology* [Internet]. 1978 Aug; 235(2): E231-6. Available from: https://pubmed.ncbi.nlm.nih.gov/686169/.

[31] Wiles CM, Jones DA, Edwards RH. Fatigue in human metabolic myopathy. *Ciba Foundation Symposium* [Internet]. 1981; 82: 264-82. Available from: https://pubmed.ncbi.nlm.nih.gov/6913475/.

[32] Zurcher RM (Berne, Switzerland), Horber FF, Grunig BE, Frey FJ. Effect of thyroid dysfunction on thigh muscle. *Journal of Clinical Endocrinology & Metabolism* [Internet]. 1989 Nov; 69(5): 1082-6. Available from: https://pubmed.ncbi.nlm.nih.gov/2793992/.

[33] Khaleeli AA, Edwards RH. Effect of treatment on skeletal muscle dysfunction in hypothyroidism. *Clinical Science* (London,

UK) [Internet]. 1984 Jan; 66(1): 63-8. Available from: https://pubmed.ncbi.nlm.nih.gov/6606523/.

[34] Ishikawa T (Nagoya, Japan), Chijiwa T, Hagiwara M, Mamiya S, Hidaka H. Thyroid hormones directly interact with vascular smooth muscle strips. *Molecular Pharmacology* [Interact]. 1989 Jun; 35(6): 760-5. Available from: https://pubmed.ncbi.nlm.nih.gov/2733694/.

[35] Ojamaa K, Balkman C, Klein IL. Acute effects of triiodothyronine on arterial smooth muscle cells [review]. *Annals of Thoracic Surgery* [Internet]. 1993 Jul; 56(1 Suppl): S61-6. Available from: https://pubmed.ncbi.nlm.nih.gov/8333799/.

[36] Ellman P. Endocrinal obesity (hypothyroidism) with oedema of the legs, osteoarthritis and hypertension. *Proceedings of the Royal Society of Medicine* [Internet]. 1938 Jun; 31(8): 918. Available from: https://www.ncbi.nlm.nih.gov/pmc/articles/PMC2076837/.

[37] Berris B (Toronto, Canada), Owen T. Unusual Manifestations of myxedema. *Canadian Medical Association Journal* [Internet]. 1965 Jul 3; 93: 21-25. Available from: https://www.ncbi.nlm.nih.gov/pmc/articles/PMC1928647/.

[38] Lerman J (Mass. Genl. Hosp., Boston, MA), Clark R, Means JH. The heart in myxedema: electrocardiograms and roentgen-ray measurements before and after therapy. *Annals of Internal Medicine* [Internet]. 1933 Apr 1; 6(10): 1251-71. Available from: https://www.acpjournals.org/doi/10.7326/0003-4819-6-10-1251.

[39] Okamura K, Inoue K, Shiroozu A, Nakashima T, Yoshinari M, Omae T, Yoshizumi T, Nishitani H. [Primary hypothyroidism as a possible cause of hypertension from long-term follow-up studies of patients with Graves' disease (author's translation)] [article in Japanese]. *Nihon Naibunpi Gakkai Zasshi* [Internet]. 1980 June 20; 56(6): 767-75. Available from: https://pubmed.ncbi.nlm.nih.gov/6893308/.

[40] Bing RF, Briggs, RS, Burden, AC, Russell GI, Swales JD, Thurston H. Reversible hypertension and hypothyroidism. *Clinical Endocrinology* (Oxf). [Internet]. 1980 Oct;13(4):339-42. Available from: https://pubmed.ncbi.nlm.nih.gov/7438475/.

[41] Saito I, Ito K, Saruta T. Hypothyroidism as a cause of hypertension [comparative study]. *Hypertension* [Internet]. 1983; 5(1): 112-5. Available from: https://pubmed.ncbi.nlm.nih.gov/6848458/.

[42] Yamamoto K, Saito K, Takai T, Yoshida S. Unusual manifestations in primary hypothyroidism [review]. *Progress in Clinical and Biological Research* [Internet]. 1983; 116: 169-87. Available from: https://pubmed.ncbi.nlm.nih.gov/6222384/.

[43] Ladenson PW, Goldenheim PD, Ridgway EC. Prediction and reversal of blunted ventilatory responsiveness in patients with hypothyroidism. *American Journal of Medicine* [Internet]. 1988 May; 84(5): 877-83. Available from: https://pubmed.ncbi.nlm.nih.gov/3364447/.

[44] Ambrosino N (Italy), Pacini F, Paggiaro PL, Martino E, Contini V, Turini L, Tarchi M, Vitti P, Bramanti M, Pinchera A. Impaired ventilatory drive in short-term primary hypothyroidism and its reversal by L-triiodothyronine. *Journal of Endocrinology Investigation* [Internet]. 1985 Dec; 8(6): 533-6. Available from: https://pubmed.ncbi.nlm.nih.gov/3833897/.

[45] Laroche CM (Brompton Hosp., London, England), Cairns T, Moxham J, Green M. Hypothyroidism presenting with respiratory muscle weakness [case report]. American Review of Respiratory Diseases [Internet]. 1988 Aug: 138(2): 472-4. Available from: https://pubmed.ncbi.nlm.nih.gov/3195839/.

[46] Siafakas NM (Heraklion, Greece), Salesiotou V, Filaditaki V, Tzanakis N, Thalassinos N, Bouros D. Respiratory muscle strength in hypothyroidism. *Chest* [Internet]. 1992 Jul; 102(1): 189-94. Available from: https://pubmed.ncbi.nlm.nih.gov/1623751/.

[47] Sadek SH (Assuit, Egypt), Khalifa WA, Azoz AH. Pulmonary consequences of hypothyroidism. *Annals of Thoracic Medicine* [Internet]. 2017 Jul-Sept; 12(3): 204-8. Available from: https://ncbi.nlm.nih.gov/pmc/articles/PMC5541969/.

[48] Peters JP (Dept of Internal Medicine, Yale University School of Medicine, New Haven, CT), Man EB. The significance of serum cholesterol in thyroid disease. *Journal of Clinical Investigation* [Internet]. 1950 Jan [Cited 2019 Oct 8]; 29(1): 1-11. Available from: https://ncbi.nlm.nih.gov/pmc/articles/pmc439718/.

[49] Turner KB. Studies on the prevention of cholesterol atherosclerosis in rabbits: 1. The effects of whole thyroid and of potassium iodide. *Journal of Experimental Medicine* [Internet]. 1933 June 30; 58(1): 115-25. Available from: https://www.ncbi.nlm.nih.gov/pubmed/19870177/.

[50] Barnes BO, Barnes CW. *Solved: The Riddle of Heart Attacks.* 6th edition. Fort Collins, CO: Robinson Press, Inc.; 1984. 74 p. Available from: The Broda Barnes Foundation; Trumbull, CT; at https://brodabarnes.org/bookstore.htm.

[51] Barnes BO, Galton L. *Hypothyroidism: the Unsuspected Illness.* New York: Harper & Row; 1976. 286 p.

[52] Hodis H. (Director, Atherosclerosis Research Unit, Univ. of Southern California, LA, CA.). Personal e-mail communication. 2019 Dec 1.

[53] Canner PL, Berge KG, Wenger NK, Stamler J, Friedman L, Prineas RJ, Friedewald W. Fifteen year mortality in Coronary Drug Project patients: long-term benefit with niacin [clinical trial]. *Journal American College of Cardiology* [Internet]. 1986 Dec; 8(6): 1245-55. Available from: https://pubmed.ncbi.nlm.nih.gov/3782631/.

[54] Miura S (Fourth Dept. of Internal Medicine, Saitama Medical School, Japan), Iitaka M, Yoshimura H, Kitahama S, Fukasawa N, Kawakami Y, Sakurai S, Urabe M, Sakatsume Y, Ito K, et al.

Disturbed lipid metabolism in patients with subclinical hypothyroidism: effect of L-thyroxine therapy [abstract]. *Internal Medicine* [Internet]. 1994 Jul; 33(7): 413-7. Available from: https://www.ncbi.nlm.nih.gov/pubmed/7949641/.

[55] Gluvic Z (Belgrade, Serbia), Sudar E, Tica J, Jovanovic A, Zafirovic S, Tomasevic R, Isenovic E. Effects of levothyroxine replacement therapy on parameters of metabolic syndrome and atherosclerosis in hypothyroid patients: a prospective pilot study. *International Journal of Endocrinology* [Internet]. 2015 Mar 2. Available from: https://www.ncbi.nlm.nih.gov/pmc/articles/PMC4363579/.

[56] Haller H. [Epidermiology and associated risk factors of hyperlipoproteinemia] [Article in German]. *Z Gesamte Inn Med.* 1977 Apr 15; 32(8): 124-8. Available from: https://pubmed.ncbi.nlm.nih.gov/883354/.

[57] Healthprep.com [Internet]. St. Michael, Barbados, WI: Pub Labs International, Inc; c 2016-2020. Treating and managing metabolic syndrome; [Cited 2019 Nov 30]. Available from: https://healthprep.com/conditions/treating-managing-metabolic-syndrome/.

[58] Starr M. *Hypothyroidism Type 2.* Columbia, MO: Mark Starr Trust; 2005. 242 p.

[59] La Mer Website, https://www.cremedelamer.com/product/20652/74983/face/eye-treatments/the-eye-concentrate.

[60] Skinpeutics website, https://skinpeutics.com.

[61] Golding DN (Princess Alexandra Hospital and Harlow Group, Hertfordshire and Essex, UK). Hypothyroidism presenting with musculoskeletal symptoms. *Annals of Rheumatologic Diseases* [Internet]. 1970; 29: 10-4. Available from: http://ncbi.nlm.nih.gov/pmc/articles/PMC1031216/.

[62] Perkins AT, Morgenlander JC. Endocrinologic causes of peripheral neuropathy. Pins and needles in a stocking-and-glove

pattern and other symptoms [abstract]. *Postgraduate Medicine* [Internet]. 1997 Sep; 102(3): 81-2, 90-2, 102-6. Available from: https://pubmed.ncbi.nlm.nih.gov/9300020/.

[63] Duyff RF (Amsterdam, The Netherlands), Van den Bosch J, Laman DM, van Loon BJ, Linssen WH. Neuromuscular findings in thyroid dysfunction: a prospective clinical and electrodiagnostic study. *Journal of Neurology Neurosurgery Psychiatry* [Internet]. 2000 Jun; 68(6): 750-5. Available from: https://pubmed.ncbi.nlm.nih.gov/10811699/.

[64] Palumbo CF, Szabo RM, Olmsted SL. The effects of hypothyroidism and thyroid replacement on the development of carpal tunnel syndrome. *Journal of Hand Surgery* [Internet]. 2000 Jul; 25(4): 734-9. Available from: https://pubmed.ncbi.nlm.nih.gov/10913216/.

[65] Tuppin P (Paris, FR), Blotiere PO, Weill A, Ricordeau P, Allemand H. [Carpal tunnel syndrome surgery in France in 2008: patients' characteristics and management] [article in French]. *Rev Neurol* (Paris) [Internet]. 2011 Dec; 16712 905-15. Available from: https://pubmed.ncbi.nlm.nih.gov/22035728/.

[66] Jha A (New Delhi, India), Sharma SK, Tandon N, Lakshmy R, Kadhiravan T, Handa KK, Gupta R, Pandey RM, Chaturvedi PK. Thyroxine replacement therapy reverses sleep-disordered breathing in patients with primary hypothyroidism. *Sleep Medicine* [Internet]. 2006 Jan; 7(1): 55-61. Available from: https://pubmed.ncbi.nlm.nih.gov/16198143/.

[67] Melville JC, Menegotto KD, Woernley TC, Maida BD, Alava I 3rd. Unusual case of a massive macroglossia secondary to myxedema: a case report and literature review. *Journal of Maxillofacial Surgery* [Internet]. 2018 Jan; 76(1): 119-27. Available from: https://pubmed.ncbi.nlm.nih.gov/28742994/.

[68] MayoClinic.org [Internet]. Mayo Foundation for Medical Education & Research: Leg swelling; [Cited 2020 May 25].

Available from: https://mayoclinic.org/symptoms/leg-swelling/basics/causes/sym-20050910.

[69] Summers VK (Walton Hospital, Liverpool, UK). Myxoedema Coma. *British Medical Journal* [Internet]. 1953 Aug 15; 2(4832): 366-368. Available from: https://pubmed.ncbi.nlm.nih.gov/13059511/.

[70] Villalba NL (Strasbourg, France), Zulfiqar AA, Saint-Mezard V, Belen Alonso Ortiz M, Kechida M, Fuertes Zamorano N, Suarez Ortega S. Myxedema coma: four patients diagnosed at the internal medicine department of the Dr. Negrin University Hospital in Spain [case series]. *Pan African Medical Journal* [Internet]. 2019; 34: 7. Available from: https://www.panafrican-med-journal.com/content/article/34/7/full/.

[71] Muller, R (Germany). [Hoarseness] [article in German]. *Ther Umsch* [Internet]. 1995 Nov; 52(11): 759-62. Available from: https://pubmed.ncbi.nlm.nih.gov/7502253/.

[72] Schwartz SR, Cohen SM, Dailey SH, Rosenfeld RM, Deutsch ES, Gillespie MB, et al. Clinical practice guideline: hoarseness (dysphonia) [practice guideline]. *Otolaryngology and Head Neck Surgery* [Internet]. 2009 Sep; 141(3 Suppl 2): S1-S31. Available from: https://pubmed.ncbi.nlm.nih.gov/19729111/.

[73] Reiter R (Munich, Germany), Hoffmann TK, Pickhard A, Brosch S. Hoarseness – causes and treatments [review]. *Dtsch Arztebl Int* [Internet]. 2015 May 8; 112(19): 329-37. Available from: https://pubmed.ncbi.nlm.nih.gov/26043420/.

[74] Wang Z. [Diagnosis and treatment in 45 patients with Hashimoto's thyroiditis associated with throat symptoms] [article in Chinese]. *Lin Chuang Er Bi Yan Hou Ke Za Zhi* [Internet]. 2003 Feb; 17(2):81-3. Available from: https://pubmed.ncbi.nlm.nih.gov/12833688/.

[75] Nejad SB, Qadim HH, Nazeman L, Fadaii R, Goldust M (Tabriz, Iran). Frequency of autoimmune diseases in those

suffering from vitiligo in comparison with normal population. *Pakistan Journal of Biological Sciences* [Internet]. 2013 Jun 15; 16(12): 570-4. Available from: https://pubmed.ncbi.nlm.nih.gov/24494526/.

[76] Jara LJ, Navarro C, Brito-Zeron MP, Garcia-Carrasco M, Escarcega RO, Ramos-Casals M (Mexico City, Mexico). Thyroid disease in Sjogren's syndrome [review]. *Clinical Rheumatology* [Internet]. 2007 Oct; 26(10): 1606-6. Available from: https://pubmed.ncbi.nlm.nih.gov/17558463/.

[77] Ebert EC. The thyroid and the gut. *Journal of Clinical Gastroenterology* [Internet]. 2010 Jul; 44(6): 402-6. Available from: https://pubmed.ncbi.nlm.nih.gov/20351569/.

[78] Pustorino S (Messina, Sicily, Italy), Foti M, Calipari G, Pustorino E, Ferraro R, Guerrisi O, Germanotta G. [Thyroid-intestinal motility interactions summary] [abstract] [article in Italian]. *Minerva Gastroenterol Dietol.* 2004 Dec; 50(4): 305-15. Available from: https://www.ncbi.nlm.nih.gov/pubmed/15788986/.

[79] MayoClinic.org [Internet]. Mayo Foundation for Medical Education & Research: c 1998-2022. Dysphagia Diagnosis and Treatment: [Cited 2020 Apr 16]. Available from: https://www.mayoclinic.org/distases-conditions/dysphagia/diagnosis-treatment/drc-20372033

[80] Pernambuco L (Universidade Federal da Paraiba, Joao Pessoa, Brasil), Silva MP, Almeida MN, Costa EB, Souza LB. Self-perception of swallowing by patients with benign nonsurgical thyroid disease [article in English, Portuguese]. *Codas* [Internet]. 2017 Feb 23; 29(1): E20160020. Available from: https://pubmed.ncbi.nlm.nih.gov/28273248/.

[81] Eastwood GL, Braverman LE, White EM, Vander Salm TJ. Reversal of lower esophageal sphincter hypotension and esophageal aperistalsis after treatment for hypothyroidism. *Journal*

of Clinical Gastroenterology [Internet]. 1982 Aug; 4(4): 307-10. Available from: https://pubmed.ncbi.nlm.nih.gov/7119407/.

[82] Urquhart AD, Rea IM, Lawson LT, Skipper M. A new complication of hypothyroid coma: neurogenic dysphagia: presentation, diagnosis, and treatment. *Thyroid* [Internet]. 2001 Jun; 11(6): 595-8. Available from: https://pubmed.ncbi.nlm.nih.gov/11442008/.

[83] Ilhan M (Dept. of Endocrinology and Metabolism, Benmialem University, Istanbul, Turkey), Arabici E, Turgut S, Karaman O, Danalioglu A, Tasan E. Esophagus motility in overt hypothyroidism. *Journal of Endocrinology investigation* [Internet]. 2014 Jul; 37(7): 639-44. Available from: https://pubmed.ncbi.nlm.nih.gov/24844564/.

[84] Kukolja K (Radna jedinica za interne bolesti Medicinski centar, Varazdin, Croatia), Dvorscak D, Beer Z, Dumicic J. [Intestinal pseudoobstruction in hypothyroidism] [abstract] [article in Croatian]. *Lijec Vjesn* [Internet]. 1990 May-Jun: 112(5-6): 165-7. Available from: https://pubmed.ncbi.nlm.nih.gov/2233114/.

[85] Fiorani S (Rome, Italy), Reda G, Cesareo R, Tomba G, Visentin PP. [Hypothyroidism and megacolon] [case report] [article in Italian*]*. *Minerva Anestesiol* [Internet]. 1996 Jul-Aug; 62(7-8): 271-5. Available from: https://pubmed.ncbi.nlm.nih.gov/8999378/.

[86] Shafer RB, Prentiss RA, Bond JH. Gastrointestinal transit in thyroid disease. *Gastroenterology* [Internet]. 1984 May; 86(5 Pt 1): 852-5. Available from: https://pubmed.ncbi.nlm.nih.gov/6706068/.

[87] Sinha RA (Laboratory of Hormonal Regulation, Cardiovascular and Metabolic Disorders Programme, Duke-NUS Medical School, Singapore), Singh BK, Yen PM. Direct effects of thyroid hormones on hepatic lipid metabolism. *National Review of Endocrinology* [Internet]. 2018 May; 14(5): 259-69. Available from: https://pubmed.ncbi.nlm.nih.gov/29472712/.

[88] MayoClinic.org [Internet]. Mayo Foundation for Medical Education & Research: c 1998-2022. Cholesterol medications: consider the options; [Cited 2020 May 26]. Available from: https://www.mayoclinic.org/diseases-conditons/high-blood-cholesterol/in-depth/cholesterol-medications/art-20050958/.

[89] WebMD.com [Internet]. WebMD, LLC; 2018. 12 Common side effects of cholesterol drugs; [Cited 2020 May 26]. Available from: https://www.webmd.com/cholesterol-management/common-side-effects-cholesterol-meds/.

[90] MayoClinic.org [Internet]. Mayo Foundation for Medical Education & Research: Nonalcoholic fatty liver disease; [Cited 2020 May 20]. Available from: https://mayoclinic.org/diseases-conditions/nonalcoholic-fatty-liver-disease/symptoms-causes/SYC-20354567/.

[91] Sinha RA (Laboratory of Hormonal Regulation, Cardiovascular and Metabolic Disorders Programme, Duke-NUS Medical School, Singapore), Singh BK, Yen PM. Direct effects of thyroid hormones on hepatic lipid metabolism. *National Review of Endocrinology* [Internet]. 2018 May; 14(5): 259-69. Available from: https://pubmed.ncbi.nlm.nih.gov/29472712/.

[92] Tsuchiya Y (Kanazawa, Japan), Nakajima M, Yokoi T. Cytochrome P450-mediated metabolism of estrogens and its regulation in human [review]. *Cancer Letters* [Internet]. 2005 Sep 28; 227(2): 115-24. Available from: https://pubmed.ncbi.nlm.nih.gov/16112414/.

[93] Wikipedia.org [Internet]. Wikimedia Foundation, Inc. Polycystic ovary syndrome; [Last edited 2022 Dec 8]; Cited 2019 Jul 21]. Available from: https://en.wikipedia.org/wiki/Polycystic_ovary_syndrome.

[94] Pubmed.gov [Internet]. Bethesda, MD: National Institutes of Health, National Library of Medicine, National Center for Biotechnology Information. Search for the phrase "Use of thyroid for fertility"; [Cited 2020 Jul 27]. Available from:

https://pubmed.ncbi.nlm.nih.gov/?term=use_of_thyroid_for_in fertility&sort=pubdate&sort_order=asc.

[95] Trokoudes KM [Pedieos IVF Center, Cyprus], Skordis N, Picolos MK. Infertility and thyroid disorders [review]. *Current Opinion Obstetrics & Gynecology* [Internet]. 2006 Aug; 18(4): 446-51. Available from: https://pubmed.ncbi.nlm.nih.gov/16794427/.

[96] Naficy H (Iran), Behjatnia Y. The effect of thyroid extract on luteal phase deficiency [comparative study]. Acta Med Iran [Internet]. 1975; 18(1-2): 55-60. Available from: https://pubmed.ncbi.nlm.nih.gov/1241836/.

[97] Natori S (Dept. of Internal Medicine, Iizuka Hospital, Japan), Karashima T, Koga S, Abe M, Tominaga K. [A case report of idiopathic myxedema with secondary amenorrhoea and hyperprolactinemia: effect of thyroid hormone replacement on reduction of pituitary enlargement and restoration of fertility] [article in Japanese] [case report]. *Fukuoka Igaku Zasshi.* 1991 Aug; 82(8): 461-3. Available from: https://pubmed.ncbi.nlm.nih.gov/1937345/.

[98] Tadmor OP (Gyn Dept., Shaare Zedek Medical Center, Jerusalem, Israel), Barr I, Diamant YZ. [Primary hypothyroidism presenting with amenorrhea, galactorrhea, hyperprolactinemia and enlarged pituitary] [article in Hebrew] [case report]. *Harefuah* [Internet]. 1992 Jan 15; 122(2): 76-8. Available from: https://www.pubmed.ncbi.nlm.nih.gov/1572562/.

[99] Abe Y (Tokia University School of Medicine, Tokyo, Japan), Momotani N. [Thyroid disease and reproduction dysfunction] [article in Japanese] [review]. *Nihon Rinsho* [Internet]. 1997 Nov; 55(11): 2984-8. Available from: https://www.pubmed.ncbi.nlm.nih.gov/9396298/.

[100] Ramprasad M (Bangalore, India), Bhattacharyya SS, Bhattacharyya A. Thyroid disorders in pregnancy. *Indian Journal of Endocrinology & Metabolism* [Internet]. 2012 Dec; 16(Suppl 2):

S167-70. Available from: https://pubmed.ncbi.nlm.nih.gov/23565370/.

[101] Negro R (Lecce, Italy), Mestman JH. Thyroid disease in pregnancy [review]. *Best Practices Research in Clinical Endocrinology & Metabolism* [Internet]. 2011 Dec; 25(6): 927-43. Available from: https://pubmed.ncbi.nlm.nih.gov/22115167/.

[102] Velasco I (Huelva, Spain), Taylor P. The role of levothyroxine in obstetric practice [review]. *Annals of Medicine* [Internet]. 2018 Feb; 50(1): 57-67. Available from: https://pubmed.ncbi.nlm.nih.gov/28972798/ and Velasco I (Huelva, Spain), Taylor P. Identifying and treating subclinical thyroid dysfunction in pregnancy: emerging controversies [review]. *European Journal of Endocrinology* [Internet]. 2018 Jan; 178(1): D1-D12. Available from: https://pubmed.ncbi.nlm.nih.gov/29070512/.

[103] Tong Z (Shenyang, Liaoning, China), Xiaowen Z, Baomin C, Aihua L, Yingying Z, Weiping T, Zhongyan S. The effect of subclinical maternal thyroid dysfunction and autoimmunity on intrauterine growth restriction: A systematic review and mean-analysis [review]. *Medicine* (Baltimore) [Internet]. 2016 May; 95(19): e3677. Available from: https://pubmed.ncbi.nlm.nih.gov/27175703/.

[104] Milanesi A, Brent GA. Management of hypothyroidism in pregnancy [review]. *Current Opinions in Endocrinology Diabetes & Obesity* [Internet]. 2011 Oct; 18(5): 304-9. Available from: https://pubmed.ncbi.nlm.nih.gov/21841481/.

[105] Sarkar D (Bihar, India). Recurrent pregnancy loss in patients with thyroid dysfunction [Internet]. *Indian Journal of Endocrinology & Metabolism*. 2012 Dec; 16(Suppl 2): S350-1. Available from: https://pubmed.ncbi.nlm.nih.gov/23565424/.

[106] Dhillon-Smith R (Birmingham, UK), Middleton LJ, Sunner KK, Cheed V, Baker K, Farrell-Carver S, et al. Levothyroxine to increase live births in euthyroid women with thyroid antibodies

trying to conceive: the TABLET RCT [review]. Southhampton (UK): *NIHR Journals Library*; 2019 Oct. Available from: https://pubmed.ncbi.nlm.nih.gov/31617987/.

[107] Kattah A, Garovic VD. Subclinical hypothyroidism and gestational hypertension: causal or coincidence? *Journal of American Society of Hypertension* [Internet]. 2016 Sep; 10990; 688-690. Available from: https://www.ncbi.nlm.nih.gov/pmc/articles/PMC5294952/.

[108] Ramtahal R (Cunupia, Trinidad & Tobago), Dhanoo A. Subclinical hypothyroidism causing hypertension in pregnancy [case report]. *Journal of American Society of Hypertension* [Internet]. 2016 Sep; 10(9): 691-3. Available from: https://pubmed.ncbi.nlm.nih.gov/27506728/.

[109] Velkeniers B (Brussels, Belgium), Van Meerhaeghe A, Poppe K, Unuane D, Tournaye H, Haentgens P. Levothyroxine treatment and pregnancy outcome in women with subclinical hypothyroidism undergoing assisted reproduction technologies: systematicc review and meta-analysis of RCTs [review]. *Human Reproduction Update* [Internet]. 2013 May-Jun; 19(3): 251-8. Available from: https://pubmed.ncbi.nlm.nih.gov/23327883/.

[110] Rao M (Kunming, China), Zeng Z, Zhou F, Wang H, Liu J, Wang R, et al. Effect of levothyroxine supplementation on pregnancy loss and preterm birth in women with subclinical hypothyroidism and thyroid autoimmunity: a systematic review and meta-analysis [meta-analysis]. *Human Reproduction Update* [Internet]. 2019 May 1; 25(3): 344-61. Available from: https://pubmed.ncbi.nlm.nih.gov/30951172/.

[111] Argatska AB (Plovdiv, Bulgaria), Nonchev BI. Postpartum thyroiditis [review]. *Folia Med (Plovdiv)* [Internet]. 2014 Jul-Sep; 56(3): 145-51. Available from: https://pubmed.ncbi.nlm.nih.gov/25434070/.

[112] Wikipedia.org [Internet]. Wikimedia Foundation, Inc. Premenstrual syndrome: [Last edited 2020 Jun 26]; [Cited 2020

July 6]. Available from: https://en.wikipedia.org/wiki/Premenstrual_syndrome.

[113] IAPMD.org [Internet]. Boston, MA: International Association for Premenstrual Disorders. World Health Organization adds premenstrual dysphoric disorder (PMDD) into the ID-11; 2019 June 14 [Cited 2020 July 12]. Available from: https://iapmd.org/position-statements-1/2019/6/11/world-health-organization-adds-premenstrual-dysphoric-disorder-pmdd-into-the-icd-11.

[114] IAPMD.org [Internet]. Boston, MA: International Association for Premenstrual Disorders. Our mission. 2019 June 14 [Cited 2020 July 12]. Available from: https://iapmd.org/about.

[115] Theravive.com [Internet]. Theravive 2006-2022. Therapedia: Premenstrual dysphoric disorder DSM-5 625.4 (N94.3); [Cited 2020 Jul 12]. Available from: https://www.theravive.com/therapedia/premenstrual-dysphoric-disorder-dsm-5-625.4-(n94.3).

[116] Daw, J. (2002). Is PMDD real? *Amer Psychol Assoc Monitor.* 33(9), 58.

[117] Stolberg, M. (2000). The monthly malady: A history of premenstrual suffering. *Med Hist,* 44, 301-322.

[118] Drugs.com [Internet]. Dallas, TX: Drugsite Ltd; 2000-2022. Progesterone Side Effects; [Cited 2020 Jul 24]. Available from: https://www.drugs.com/sfx/progesterone-side-effects.html.

[119] DoveMed.com [Internet]. Champaign, IL: Dovemed; 2011-2022. First Aid for Estrogen Overdose; Last updated 2018 Feb 24 [Cited 2020 Jul 24]. Available from: https://www.dovemed.com/healthy-living/first-aid/first-aid-estrogen-overdose/.

[120] Barnes BO, Galton L. *Hypothyroidism: the Unsuspected Illness. New York*: Harper & Row; 1976. 286 p.

[121] Nikolai TF, Mulligan GM, Gribble RK, Harkins PG, Meier PR, Roberts RC. Thyroid function and treatment in premenstrual syndrome. *Journal Clinical Endocrinology & Metabolism* [Internet]. 1990 Apr; 70(4): 1108-13. Available from: https://pubmed.ncbi.nlm.nih.gov/2108182/.

[122] Zaproudina N, Lipponen JA, Karjalainen PA, Kamshilin AA, Giniatullin R, Narhi M (Kuopio, Finland). Acral coldness in migraineurs. *Autonomic Neuroscience: Basic & Clinical* [Internet]. 2014 Feb; 80: 70-3. Available from: https://www.autonomicneuroscience.com/article/S1566-0702(13)00702-9/abstract.

[123] New York Headache Blog. Available from: https://www.nyheadache.com/blog/cold-hands-and-nose-in-migraine-sufferers/.

[124] HealthSoul.com [Internet]. Phoenix, AZ. Cretinism: symptoms, causes and treatment [blog]; 2018 Jul 26 [Cited 2019 Aug 4]. Available from: https://healthsoul.com/blog/cretinism-symptoms-causes-and-treatment/.

[125] ScienceDirect.com [Internet]. Elsevier BV. Iodine deficiency [publication list].; 2022 [Cited 2019 Aug 4]. Available from: https://www.sciencedirect.com/search?qs=iodine%20deficiency.

[126] NIH National Institute of Neurological Disorders and Stroke [Internet]. Bethesda, MD; National Institutes of Health, NINDS, Office of Communications & Public Liaison. Brain basics: understanding sleep; [Last reviewed 2022 Apr 1; Cited 2022 Jul 12]. Available from: https://www.ninds.nih.gov/health-information/patient-caregiver-education/brain-basics-understanding-sleep.

[127] Wang H, Tan Z, Zheng Q, Yu J (Dalian, Liaoning, China). Metabolic brain network analysis of hypothyroidism symptom based on [18F] FDG-PET of rats [abstract]. *Molecular Imaging Biology* [Internet]. 2018 Oct; 20(5): 789-97. Available from: https://pubmed.ncbi.nlm.nih.gov/29532350/.

[128] Skinner GRB. *Diagnosis and Management of Hypothyroidism.* Biggleswade, UK: Watkiss Studios, Ltd.; 2003. 199 p.

[129] Kelly C, McCreadie R. Cigarette smoking and schizophrenia. *British Journal of Psych Advances,* Advances in Psychiatric Treatment [Internet]. 2000 Sept: 6(5); 327-31). Available from: https://www.cambridge.org/core/journals/advances-in-psychiatric-treatment/article/cigarette-smoking-and-schizophrenia/AF9CC53E7777F37A8FF6E27F4336DBEE#.

[130] Barnes BO, Galton L. *Hypothyroidism: the Unsuspected Illness.* New York: Harper & Row; 1976. 286 p.

[131] Moley JF, Ohkawa M, Chaudry IH, Clemens MG Baue AE. Hypothyroidism abolishes the hyperdynamic phase and increases susceptibility to sepsis. *Journal of Surgery Research* [Internet]. 1984 Mar; 36(3): 265-73. Available from: https://pubmed.ncbi.nlm.nih.gov/6700215/.

[132] Barnes BO, Barnes CW. *Solved: The Riddle of Heart Attacks.* 6th edition. Fort Collins, CO: Robinson Press, Inc.; 1984. 74 p. Available from The Broda Barnes Foundation; Trumbull, CT; at https://brodabarnes.org/bookstore.htm.

[133] Tan TL, Rajeswaran H, Haddad S, Shahi A, Parvizi J. Increased risk of periprosthetic joint infections in patients with hypothyroidism undergoing total joint arthroplasty. *Journal of Arthroplasty* [Internet]. 2016 Apr; 31(4): 868-71. Available from: https://pubmed.ncbi.nlm.nih.gov/26777546/.

[134] Liu WK (Chinese University of Hong Kong, Sah tin, New Territories), Ng TB. Effect of methimazole-induced hypothyroidism on alveolar macrophages. *Virchows Arch B Cell Pathol Incl Mol Pathol* [Internet]. 1991; 60(1): 21-6. Available from: https://pubmed.ncbi.nlm.nih.gov/1673273/.

[135] Hodkinson CF, Simpson EE, Beattie JH, O'Connor JM, Campbell DJ, Strain JJ, Wallace JM. Preliminary evidence of immune function modulation by thyroid hormones in healthy

men and women aged 50-70 years. *Journal of Endocrinology* [Internet]. 2009 Jul; 202(1): 55-63. Available from: https://pubmed.ncbi.nlm.nih.gov/19398496/

[136] Papaioannou G (Athens, Greece), Michelis FV, Papamichael K, Karga H, Tiligada K. Blood lymphocyte blastogenesis in patients with thyroid dysfunction: ex vivo response to mitogen activation and cyclosporin A. *Inflammation Research* [Internet]. 2011 Mar; 60(3): 265-70. Available from: https://pubmed.ncbi.nlm.nih.gov/20972816/.

[137] De Vito, P (Rome, Italy), Incerpi S, Pedersen JZ, Luly P, Davis FB, Davis PJ. Thyroid hormones as modulators of immune activities at the cellular level [review]. *Thyroid* [Internet]. 2011 Aug; 21(8): 879-90. Available from: https://pubmed.ncbi.nlm.nih.gov/21745103/.

[138] Burrell C. Elderly cope with 'the dwindles'. *Los Angeles Times* (internet edition). 1995 Jun 18 [Cited 2020 Aug 4]. Available from: https://www.latimes.com/archives/la-xpm-1995-06-18-mn-14558-story.html.

[139] Brokhin M, Danzi S, Klein I. Assessment of the adequacy of thyroid hormone replacement therapy in hypothyroidism. *Frontiers in Endocrinology* (Lausanne, Switzerland) [Internet]. 2019 Sep 20; 10 (631): 1-7. Available from: https://ncbi.nlm.nih.gov/pmc/articles/PMC6763555/.

[140] Billewicz WZ, Chapman RS, Crooks J, Day ME, Gossage J, Wayne E, et al. Statistical methods applied to the diagnosis of hypothyroidism. *Quarterly Journal of Medicine*. 1969 Apr; 38(150): 255-66. Available from: https://academic.oup.com/qjmed/article-abstract/38/2/255/1589928/.

[141] www.NAhypothyroidism.org [Internet]. National Academy of Hypothyroidism. 2012-2022 [Cited 2022 May 23]. Available from: https://www.nahypothyroidism.org/about/.

[142] NAhypothyroidism.org [Internet]. National Academy of Hypothyroidism; 2012-2022. How accurate is TSH testing? 2012 Jan 27 [Cited 2021 May 23]. Available from: https://www.nahypothyroidism.org/how-accurate-is-tsh-testing/.

[143] Zulewski H (Basel, Switzerland), Muller B, Exer P, Miserez AR, Staub JJ. Estimation of tissue hypothyroidism by a new clinical score: Evaluation of patients with various grades of hypothyroidism and controls. *Journal of Clinical Endocrinology & Metabolism* [Internet]. 1997 Mar; 82(3): 771-6. Available from: https://pubmed.ncbi.nlm.nih.gov/9062480/.

[144] NAhypothyroidism.org [Internet]. National Academy of Hypothyroidism; 2012-2022. Why doesn't my endocrinologist know all of this? 2012 Jan 27 [Cited 2021 May 23]. Available from: https://nahypothyroidism.org/why-doesnt-my-doctor-know-all-of-this/.

[145] Goodreads.com [Internet]. Goodreads, Inc, Otis Chandler, 2007-2022. Daniel J. Boorstin>quotes>quotable quote [Cited 2022 July 20]. Available from: https://www.goodreads.com/quotes/560795-the-greatest-obstacle-to-discovering-the-shape-of-the-earth

[146] Skinner GRB. *Diagnosis and Management of Hypothyroidism.* Biggleswade, UK: Watkiss Studios, Ltd.; 2003. 199 p.

[147] Thicke, Robin; Williams, Pharrell; Harris, Clifford; Gaye, Marvin; composers. "Blurred Lines." *Blurred Lines (album)*, performance by Robin Thicke, Pharrell Williams and TI. Startrak: Interscope. 2013.

[148] Healthgrades.com [Internet]. Denver & Atlanta: Healthgrades Marketplace, LLC.; 1998-2022. The top 50 drugs prescribed in the United States; Lewis, Sarah; 2019 Sep 5 [Cited 2020 Dec 8]. Available from: https://www.healthgrades.com/right-care/patient-advocate/the-top-50-drugs-prescribed-in-the-united-states.

[149] Brokhin M, Danzi S, Klein I. Assessment of the adequacy of thyroid hormone replacement therapy in hypothyroidism. *Frontiers in Endocrinology* (Lausanne, Switzerland) [Internet]. 2019 Sep 20; 10 (631): 1-7. Available from: https://ncbi.nlm.nih.gov/pmc/articles/PMC6763555/.

[150] Billewicz WZ, Chapman RS, Crooks J, Day ME, Gossage J, Wayne E, et al. Statistical methods applied to the diagnosis of hypothyroidism. *Quarterly Journal of Medicine*. 1969 Apr; 38(150): 255-66. Available from: https://academic.oup.com/qjmed/article-abstract/38/2/255/1589928/.

[151] Zulewski H (Basel, Switzerland), Muller B, Exer P, Miserez AR, Staub JJ. Estimation of tissue hypothyroidism by a new clinical score: Evaluation of patients with various grades of hypothyroidism and controls. *Journal of Clinical Endocrinology & Metabolism* [Internet]. 1997 Mar; 82(3): 771-6. Available from: https://pubmed.ncbi.nlm.nih.gov/9062480/.

[152] Tenenbein M, Dean HJ. Benign course after massive levothyroxine ingestion. *Pediatric Emergency Care* [Internet]. 1986 Mar; 2(1): 15-7. Available from: https://pubmed.ncbi.nlm.nih.gov/3774567/.

[153] Gorman RL (Univ. of Maryland School of Pharmacy, Baltimore, MD.), Chamberlain JM, Rose SR, Oderda GM. Massive levothyroxine overdose: high anxiety – low toxicity [case report]. Available from: https://pubmed.ncbi.nlm.nih.gov/3174321/.

[154] Nystrom E, Lindstedt G, Lundberg PA. Minor signs and symptoms of toxicity in a young woman in spite of massive thyroxine ingestion [case report]. *Acta Med Scand* [Internet]. 1980; 207(1-2): 135-6. Available from: https://pubmed.ncbi.nlm.nih.gov/7368967/.

[155] Matthews SJ (Royal Victoria Hospital, Belfast, Ireland). Acute thyroxine overdosage: two cases of parasuicide [review]. *Ulster*

Med J. [Internet]. 1993 Oct; 62(2): 170-3. Available from: https://pubmed.ncbi.nlm.nih.gov/7905687/.

[156] Hofe SE, Young RL. Thyrotoxicosis after a single ingestion of levothyroxine [case report*]. Journal of the American Medical Association* [Internet]. 1977 Mar 28; 237(13): 1361. Available from: https://pubmed.ncbi.nlm.nih.gov/576486/.

[157] Nygaard B (Copenhagen University Hospital, Bispejerg, Denmark), Saedder EA, Dalhoff K, Wikkelsoe M, Jurgens G. Levothyroxine poisoning – symptoms and clinical outcome. *Basic & Clinical Pharmacology & Toxicology* [Internet]. 2015; 117: 280-5. Available from: https://onlinelibrary.wiley.com/doi/10.1111/bcpt.12401.

[158] Lobo RA, Pickar JH, Stevenson JC, Mack WJ, Hodis HN. Back to the future: hormone replacement therapy as part of a prevention strategy for women at the onset of menopause [review]. *Atherosclerosis* [Internet]. 2016 Nov; 254: 282-290. Available from: https://pubmed.ncbi.nlm.nih.gov/27745704/.

[159] StopTheThyroidMadness.com [Internet]. 2005-2022. Janie's Blog – Very sad news: Dr Gordon P. Skinner of the UK has passed away! 2013 Nov 28 [Cited 2021 Mar 10]. Available from: https://stopthethyroidmadness.com/2013/11/28/gordon-skinner/.

[160] Chahardoli R (Tehran, Iran), Saboor-Yaraghi AA, Amouzegar A, Khalili D, Vakili AZ, Azizi F. Can supplementation with vitamin D modify thyroid autoantibodies (anti-TPO ab, anti-Tg ab) and thyroid profile (T3, T4, TSH) in Hashimoto's thyroiditis? A double blind, randomized clinical trial [randomized controlled trial]. *Hormone Metabolism Research* [Internet]. 2019 May; 51(5): 296-310. Available from: https://pubmed.ncbi.nlm.nih.gov/31071734/.

[161] Holick MA. *The vitamin D solution: a 3-step strategy to cure our most common health problems.* Paperback, illustrated edition. NYC: Plume, Penguin Books, Inc; 2011 Feb 22. 336 p.

[162] Meurer LN, Lena S. Cancer recurrence and mortality in women using hormone replacement therapy: meta-analysis. *Journal of Family Practice* [Internet]. 2002 Dec; 51(12): 1056-62. Available from: https://pubmed.ncbi.nlm.nih.gov/12540332/.